Handbook of Palliative Radiation Therapy

T0297059

Handbook of Palliative Radiation Therapy

Editors

Candice Johnstone, MD, MPH
Medical Director, F&MCW Cancer Network
Associate Professor, Department of Radiation Oncology
Medical College of Wisconsin
Milwaukee, Wisconsin

Stephen T. Lutz, MD, MS
Attending Radiation Oncologist
Blanchard Valley Regional Cancer Center
Findlay, Ohio

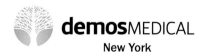

demosMEDICAL

New York

Visit our website at www.demosmedical.com

ISBN: 9781620700952
e-book ISBN: 9781617052712

Acquisitions Editor: David D'Addona
Compositor: diacriTech

Medicine is an ever-changing science. Research and clinical experience are continually expanding our knowledge, in particular our understanding of proper treatment and drug therapy. The authors, editors, and publisher have made every effort to ensure that all information in this book is in accordance with the state of knowledge at the time of production of the book. Nevertheless, the authors, editors, and publisher are not responsible for errors or omissions or for any consequences from application of the information in this book and make no warranty, expressed or implied, with respect to the contents of the publication. Every reader should examine carefully the package inserts accompanying each drug and should carefully check whether the dosage schedules mentioned therein or the contraindications stated by the manufacturer differ from the statements made in this book. Such examination is particularly important with drugs that are either rarely used or have been newly released on the market.

Library of Congress Cataloging-in-Publication Data

Names: Johnstone, Candice, editor. | Lutz, Stephen T., editor.
Title: Handbook of palliative radiation therapy / editors, Candice Johnstone, MD, MPH, Medical
   Director, F&MCW Cancer Network; and Associate Professor, Department of Radiation Oncology,
   Medical College of Wisconsin, Milwaukee, Wisconsin, Stephen T. Lutz, MD, MS, Attending
   Radiation Oncologist, Blanchard Valley Regional Cancer Center, Findlay, Ohio.
Description: New York : Demos Medical, [2017] | Includes bibliographical references and index.
Identifiers: LCCN 2016028792 | ISBN 9781620700952 | ISBN 9781617052712 (ebook)
Subjects: LCSH: Cancer—Palliative treatment—Handbooks, manuals, etc. | Cancer—Radiotherapy—
   Handbooks, manuals, etc.
Classification: LCC RC271.P33 H358 2017 | DDC 616.99/4029—dc23 LC record available at
   https://lccn.loc.gov/2016028792

Special discounts on bulk quantities of Demos Medical Publishing books are available to corporations, professional associations, pharmaceutical companies, health care organizations, and other qualifying groups. For details, please contact:
Special Sales Department
Demos Medical Publishing
11 West 42nd Street, 15th Floor, New York, NY 10036
Phone: 800-532-8663 or 212-683-0072; Fax: 212-941-7842
E-mail: specialsales@demosmedical.com

Printed in the United States of America by Publishers' Graphics.
16 17 18 19 20 / 5 4 3 2 1

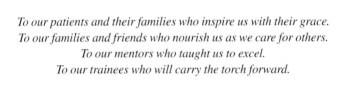

To our patients and their families who inspire us with their grace.
To our families and friends who nourish us as we care for others.
To our mentors who taught us to excel.
To our trainees who will carry the torch forward.

Contents

Contributors

Sarah Baker, MD   Chief Resident, Department of Radiation Oncology, University of Alberta, Cross Cancer Institute, Edmonton, Alberta, Canada

Nicholas Chiu, MD(c)   Medical Student, Department of Radiation Oncology, Sunnybrook Odette Cancer Centre, University of Toronto, Toronto, Ontario, Canada

Edward Chow, MBBS, MSc, PhD   Radiation Oncologist; Professor, Department of Radiation Oncology, Sunnybrook Odette Cancer Centre, University of Toronto, Toronto, Ontario, Canada

June Corry, MD, MBBS, FRACP, FRANZCR   Associate Professor, Department of Radiation Oncology, GenesisCare, St Vincents Hospital, Melbourne, Victoria, Australia

Kavita V. Dharmarajan, MD, MSc   Assistant Professor, Department of Radiation Oncology and Palliative Medicine, Icahn School of Medicine at Mount Sinai, New York, New York

Alysa Fairchild, MD, FRCPC   Associate Professor, Department of Radiation Oncology, University of Alberta, Cross Cancer Institute, Edmonton, Alberta, Canada

Sushmita Ghoshal, MD, Dip. NB   Professor and Head, Department of Radiotherapy, Regional Cancer Centre, Post Graduate Institute of Medical Education and Research, Chandigarh, India

Mohammad Hasan, MD   Radiation Oncology Resident, Department of Radiation Oncology, Sunnybrook Odette Cancer Centre, University of Toronto, Toronto, Ontario, Canada

Peter J. Hoskin, MD, FRCP, FRCR, FACR   Professor of Clinical Oncology, Consultant Clinical Oncologist, Mount Vernon Cancer Centre, Northwood; and University College London, London, UK

Candice Johnstone, MD, MPH   Medical Director, F&MCW Cancer Network; Associate Professor, Department of Radiation Oncology, Medical College of Wisconsin, Milwaukee, Wisconsin

Pei Shuen Lim, MBBS, MRCP   Clinical Oncology Specialist Registrar, Mount Vernon Cancer Centre, Northwood, UK

Raviteja Miriyala, MD Senior Resident, Department of Radiotherapy, Regional Cancer Centre, Post Graduate Institute of Medical Education and Research, Chandigarh, India

Bhavana Rai, MD, Dip. NB Assistant Professor, Department of Radiotherapy, Regional Cancer Centre, Post Graduate Institute of Medical Education and Research, Chandigarh, India

Srinivas Raman, MD, MASc Resident, Department of Radiation Oncology, Sunnybrook Odette Cancer Centre, University of Toronto, Toronto, Ontario, Canada

Jared R. Robbins, MD Assistant Professor, Department of Radiation Oncology, Medical College of Wisconsin, Milwaukee, Wisconsin

Albert Tiong, MBBS, M.App.Epi., FRANZCR Radiation Oncologist, Department of Radiation Oncology, Peter MacCallum Cancer Centre, Melbourne, Victoria, Australia

May N. Tsao, MD, FRCPC Radiation Oncologist, Department of Radiotherapy, Sunnybrook Odette Cancer Centre, University of Toronto, Toronto, Ontario, Canada

Randy Li-Hung Wei, MD, PhD Chief Resident Physician, Department of Radiation Oncology, UC Irvine School of Medicine, Orange, California

Na Zhang, MD, PhD Radiation Oncologist, Department of Radiation Oncology, Cancer Hospital of China Medical University, Liaoning Cancer Hospital & Institute, Shenyang, Liaoning, China

Preface

When people think about death and dying, they sometimes fear uncontrolled symptoms more than death itself. One common sentiment expressed in our practices is that people do not want to die in pain. Yet, many of our patients resist palliative care referrals with thoughts that "it means I am going to die" or that "I'll have to stop treatment." In the media, palliative care is often inaccurately associated with "death panels" and withholding care, something most people understandably want to avoid.

Palliative care does not accelerate death, and, in fact, seeks to enhance quality of life by relieving the physical symptoms and existential suffering associated with advanced illnesses such as cancer. Radiation therapy (RT) plays a key role in the palliation of physical symptoms due to advanced cancer.

This Work arose from a deep commitment to palliative care and in particular, palliative radiation therapy. During my tenure at my first faculty position, which was in a rural area, patients often traveled 1–2 hours to our center for radiation therapy. The need to optimize convenience for patients with severe symptoms led me to evaluate the data supporting hypofractionated or single fraction radiation therapy in a new light. Palliative RT patients need the shortest, most effective regimen to minimize travel time spent with pain, nausea, or exhaustion.

Twenty-five randomized trials have demonstrated equal pain relief between the delivery of a single fraction and multiple fractions of radiation therapy. Equivalence has been demonstrated in duration of palliative effect, time to onset of relief, complete response rates and partial response rates. Retreatment can be undertaken safely in patients who do not respond to single fraction RT. Exceptions to the absolute equivalence of single fraction radiation may include spinal cord compression or treatment of oligometastatic disease. Single fraction RT is more cost-effective and convenient for patients, yet it remains underutilized, accounting for ~ 5–7% of radiation regimens for painful bone metastasis in the United States.

During that time, I was fortunate to have found a mentor equally passionate about hypofractionated radiation in the treatment of patients with advanced cancer—my coeditor, Steve Lutz. Steve has been part of a core group of radiation oncologists promulgating hypofractionated radiation therapy for decades. He has helped formulate and promulgate guidelines for the appropriate treatment of bone metastases,[1,2] locally advanced lung cancer,[3] and glioblastoma multiforme. Steve has inspired innumerable radiation oncologists by his tireless advocacy and mentorship. His efforts led to the foundation of the Society for Palliative Radiation Oncology (SPRO) dedicated to advocacy, education, and research.

Undoubtedly, the financing of medicine in the United States, and specifically the way in which RT is reimbursed, has contributed to the use of longer courses. Yet, we also truly believe that most people, having been trained to prescribe longer courses of radiation, have trouble leaving their comfort zone and using techniques that they haven't learned about in as much detail. That is where this Work comes in—it is meant to be an extremely practical guide for physicians who want to implement shorter courses of radiation, where appropriate, into their clinical practice.

It comes at a time when the Centers for Medicare and Medicaid Services (CMS) have pledged to tie an increasing proportion of payments to value and quality.[4] Recently, CMS launched the Oncology Care Model, a pilot program targeting increasing quality and reducing costs in the care of cancer patients receiving chemotherapy.[5] Given the equivalent palliation and cost effectiveness, single fraction radiation regimens for the treatment of uncomplicated bone metastasis and hypofractionated palliative radiation regimens for other indications will likely play a key role in these settings.

Candice Johnstone, MD, MPH
Stephen T. Lutz, MD, MS

REFERENCES

1. Lutz ST, Lo SS, Chang EL, et al. ACR Appropriateness Criteria® non-spine bone metastases. *J Palliat Med*. May 2012;15(5):521-526. PubMed PMID: 22536988. Epub 2012/04/28. eng.
2. Lutz S, Berk L, Chang E, et al. Palliative radiotherapy for bone metastases: An ASTRO evidence-based guideline. *Int J Radiat Oncol Biol Phys*. March 2011;79(4):965-976. PubMed PMID: 21277118. Epub 2011/02/01. eng.
3. Rodrigues G, Videtic GM, Sur R, et al. Palliative thoracic radiotherapy in lung cancer: An American Society for Radiation Oncology evidence-based clinical practice guideline. *Pract Radiat Oncol*. April 2011;1(2):60-71. PubMed PMID: 24174996. Pubmed Central PMCID: 3808743.
4. https://www.cms.gov/Outreach-and-Education/Outreach/FFSProvPartProg/Downloads/2015-01-29-Message.pdf
5. https://innovation.cms.gov/initiatives/oncology-care/

Handbook of Palliative Radiation Therapy

1 Introduction

Candice Johnstone

Cancer is a global problem with an estimated 14.1 million new cancer cases worldwide, 32.6 million people living with cancer, and 8.2 million cancer deaths in 2012.[1] Thus, the need for good palliative care (PC) is also increasing globally as patients with advanced cancer require a coordinated multidisciplinary PC effort.

There are two fundamental categories of palliative caregivers: (a) generalist and (b) specialist. Every person who provides health care to patients with cancer or other serious illnesses should be considered a generalist and should have a comfort level with the fundamentals of PC. These fundamentals include talking with a patient to understand their goals, devising a treatment or supportive care plan consistent with those goals, management of commonly encountered symptoms and discussions about life expectancy and care at the end of life (EOL). Specialists are clinicians that have completed a PC fellowship or have additional certification in PC. They help manage refractory symptoms, navigate difficult or complex family dynamics, and help patients evaluate existential distress.[2]

PC aims to reduce pain and suffering, facilitate discussions of goals of care and death with dignity, promote quality of life, and support patients, their families, and their caregivers. The assessment includes pain and symptom assessment as well as an assessment of the social and spiritual context. Patients whose spirituality is supported by the medical team have experienced better outcomes and quality-of-life.[3–5] One commonly cited barrier noted by medical practitioners is the lack of training about how to provide such care.[6] PC providers can learn to incorporate discussions of religion and spirituality into the care that they deliver to support the spiritual needs of the patients they care for.[7] Simple acronyms, such as FICA,[7] help facilitate these conversations.

F represents faith, belief or meaning, I stands for importance and influence, C for community, and A represents address or action in care. This tool allows the health care team to determine if there is a particular faith or set of beliefs that provides meaning for a patient, assess how this faith or spirituality affects that person's life, their coping skills and decision making. This discussion can then be incorporated into subsequent care (Table 1.1).

TABLE 1.1 FICA Spiritual History Tool

FICA Spiritual History Tool		
F	Faith, belief or meaning	Do you have faith? What gives your life meaning?
I	Importance	Do these beliefs help you cope or make decisions?
C	Community	Do you belong to a community?
A	Address or action	Health care team incorporates this knowledge

Prognostication and accurate estimates of life expectancy are essential for goal setting and appropriate treatment selection. Increasingly, quality metrics surrounding the appropriate use of aggressive therapies are being developed. Avoidance of radiation therapy (RT), especially long-courses of RT, at the very EOL is important given the time course of the palliative effect of radiation. Whenever possible, the shortest course of RT likely to have the desired effect should be employed. This maximizes patient comfort and convenience and minimizes cost and toxicity.[8,9]

RT plays a key role in the palliation of physical symptoms caused by advanced cancer and serves as an adjunct to systemic analgesics, chemotherapy, interventional procedures, and supportive care. As such, radiation oncologists are essential members of a multidisciplinary PC team.

In a world of evidence-based practice and cost consciousness, physicians will increasingly utilize single fraction and short-course external beam palliative radiation courses. These approaches are critical parts of the practicing physician's knowledge base as they are generally equally efficacious, more convenient for patients, and more cost-effective.

Twenty-five randomized trials have demonstrated the equivalence of single fraction palliative radiation to longer, more expensive courses of therapy in the treatment of uncomplicated bone metastases, yet this approach is infrequently used. Single fraction RT has been hailed as a quality metric and singled out as part of the "Choosing Wisely" campaign. Similarly, in other clinical situations, there is a body of literature demonstrating equivalence of shorter courses of therapy. These approaches are more convenient for patients, many of whom have discomfort during transport.

As our health care economy moves more toward value-based care, more physicians will likely prescribe shorter courses of palliative radiation. In addition, if physicians or hospitals are reimbursed for an episode of care rather than a fee for service they will look to decrease the cost of a course of RT and utilize more cost-effective, shorter radiation regimens.

Barriers to implementation of short course and single fraction therapies include a lack of knowledge about the evidence supporting these approaches, the lack of familiarity with evaluating plans utilizing higher dose per fraction RT, and early experience using high-dose per fraction for curative therapies where the long-term toxicity proved excessive. Many physicians have never prescribed hypofractionated palliative radiation as economic incentives in the United States have long favored multifraction radiation regimens. Thus, many trainees have never been exposed to the practice. In addition, in the early days of RT, higher dose per fraction of radiation was associated with significant late complications. This is generally due to the use of large fractions in patients treated with curative intent without adjustment of the total dose of radiation to minimize late toxicity. Thus, patient selection and life expectancy are critical to the use of short course or hypofractionated palliative RT.

LIFE EXPECTANCY AND PROGNOSTICATION

Questions about life expectancy and the quality of that remaining life are extremely important to patients with metastatic cancer. Physicians and other health care providers often provide overly optimistic estimates of survival; these estimates often differ from actual survival by 3 months or more.[10] Accurate estimates of life expectancy help patients set appropriate goals, avoid futile treatments, and choose supportive care or treatments that will be effective within their remaining lifetimes.

Several themes emerge from the existent prognostication literature. Clinical predictions generally overestimate survival, but improve with repeated encounters. The patient's Karnofsky performance score is the strongest predictor of life expectancy, but other clinical factors help predict actual estimates of survival. Very poor prognostic factors include the presence of the symptom cluster known as the terminal syndrome (dyspnea, dysphagia, dry mouth, anorexia, and weight loss) or the presence of cognitive failure or confusion.[11]

Several tools were developed in the palliative RT setting and are detailed in Chapter 2 and Appendix B details tools developed in other settings. Some are easier to utilize and are more generalizable than others. The best use of these tools may be in deciding which patients may not live long enough to see the benefit of a particular treatment, since RT typically takes several days to a few weeks for its palliative effect to be seen. Patients with an extremely short life expectancy with hemoptysis and spinal cord compression may still benefit from RT as hemostasis can occur within 24 to 48 hours and the functional decline associated with spinal cord compression may significantly impair quality of life. Administration of chemotherapy within the last month of life has been promulgated as a metric of overutilization of health care.[9,10] Similar metrics may follow for RT.[12]

PALLIATIVE RT

External beam RT is a key component of palliative cancer care. It is useful to treat pain due to osseous metastasis or local tumor invasion, bleeding, obstruction, dyspnea, or cough, and functional impairment due to brain metastasis or impingement of nerve roots or the spinal cord.

Key in the utilization of RT is the selection of the shortest fractionation regimen that is effective to maximize patient and caregiver convenience and minimize toxicity and cost.[13–16] See Appendix A for fractionation schemes based on life expectancy.

Though many believe that longer courses of RT in the treatment of bone metastasis have a more durable effect, there is no data to support this belief. In the Radiation Therapy Oncology Group (RTOG) 97–14 randomized trial of fractionation, only patients with a long expected survival were enrolled. There was no difference in efficacy between 8 Gy in a single fraction and 30 Gy in 10 fractions.[13] Similarly, in an analysis of those patients who survived more than 52 weeks in the Dutch Bone Metastasis Study, there was no difference in response rate, time to response, duration of response, and time to progression of pain.[17] Randomized trials have confirmed the equivalence of short courses of RT in lung cancer[18–20] and bladder cancer,[21] and hypofractionated radiation regimens have been successfully used to treat gynecologic, gastrointestinal, and head and neck malignancies.[15]

This handbook aims to familiarize the reader with the literature supporting the use of palliative RT in various settings, and to provide a detailed guide to radiation planning and choice of fractionation with illustrative pictures and case presentations. There will be an emphasis on short course or hypofractionated approaches when appropriate.

Efficacy of palliative RT

RT provides effective pain relief in the vast majority of patients with few side effects. RT can decrease the need for systemic analgesia and can be extremely useful in patients who are intolerant of opioid analgesics.[22]

The time course for pain relief after the delivery of RT is variable and is generally not immediate. Some patients experience relief within a few days or a week of treatment but the full palliative benefit may not be evident for 4 to 6 weeks. Patients with a life expectancy less than 30 days may not benefit from RT and alternative palliative therapies should be explored. Since RT requires immobilization during treatment delivery, patients must have adequate pain relief prior to the initiation of therapy. The World Health Organization (WHO) guide to analgesia includes nonsteroidal anti-inflammatory agents, narcotic analgesics, or adjuvant pain medicines, such as corticosteroids, nerve-stabilizing medicines, or antidepressants.[23]

RT palliates other local tumor symptoms with varying frequencies. Bleeding from lung tumors can be palliated in 80% to 90% of patients. Bleeding from sources such as the stomach, bladder, uterus, and rectum can also be palliated. More complex thoracic symptoms such as cough and dyspnea are palliated with radiation but with lower rates of success. Cough and dyspnea are palliated in 60% to 90% and 40% to 60% of patients, respectively.[24–29] Symptoms associated with locally advanced gynecologic or bladder cancers are palliated in 60% to 94% of patients.[30,31] More details about the efficacy of palliative radiation in various settings are addressed in the chapters that follow.

Side effects of RT

Since the goal of palliative radiation is to relieve suffering, most palliative radiation regimens are well tolerated and designed to have few acute or long-term side effects. Acute side effects are generally mild and managed with conservative measures. With the exception of fatigue, they relate to the organs within the boundaries of the radiation field. The primary systemic side effect of radiation is fatigue. Local side effects include skin irritation, nausea, diarrhea, esophagitis, and mucositis. The total dose of radiation and the fraction size correlate with treatment toxicity. Side effects occur acutely, subacutely, or in the long-term.

By definition, late effects occur several months to years after RT. They are generally rare and irreversible. There is a correlation between a higher fraction size and the risk of late effects, though established palliative regimens have very low rates of serious late effects. Patients with advanced cancer typically do not survive long enough to be at significant risk for the development of serious late complications of RT. Improvements in systemic therapies may ultimately increase the expected survival for patients with advanced cancer and thus place them at risk of late complications that can be associated with higher daily doses of radiation. Given the modest total doses employed and the relatively limited life spans of patients with metastatic cancer, this has not been a significant problem.

GUIDELINES AND QUALITY MEASURES

The overwhelming evidence from multiple randomized trials suggests equivalence between single and multifraction approaches with increased cost and inconvenience associated with multifraction RT. More than 101 different dose regimens have been employed worldwide for this single clinical circumstance.[32] Both the American Society for Radiation Oncology (ASTRO) and the American College of Radiology (ACR) have guidelines for the

TABLE 1.2 Single Fraction RT Utilization

	Percentage of Single Fraction RT
Medicare Prostate Cancer[39]	3.3
National Cancer Database[42]	7.4
Johns Hopkins[40]	7.6
Ontario[38]	44
British Columbia[41]	49

treatment of uncomplicated bone metastasis with four approved, equivalent fractionation schemes (8 Gy/1 fraction, 20 Gy/4 fractions, 24 Gy/6 fractions, and 30 Gy/10 fractions).[33–35] The National Quality Forum (NQF) has established the use of one of these four fractionation schemes as a quality metric.[36] The American Board of Internal Medicine's "Choosing Wisely" campaign, a program designed to help physicians become better financial stewards of health care use, designates single fraction RT as the treatment of choice for painful uncomplicated bone metastasis.[37] Table 1.2 lists the percentage of single fraction RT utilized in various clinical settings. There is great variability between locations and between physicians in a given practice location.[38–42]

Two Canadian provinces attempted interventions to increase the use of single fraction RT. In Ontario, a provincial practice guideline was introduced in 2004. The use of single fraction RT increased to 53% in the 3 years following the guideline introduction but then reverted to the preguideline level of 44% during 2009 to 2012.[38–42] In British Columbia, an identified regional cancer center with anonymous physician level data was presented to all radiation oncologists in 2012. The use of single fraction RT for bone metastasis increased from a baseline of 48% to 50% to 60%. It is not yet known whether this increase was sustained.[43]

END OF LIFE RADIATION THERAPY

Chemotherapy administration in the last month of life has been recommended as a metric of resource overutilization.[8] A similar RT metric may be the use of RT in the last 2 weeks of life as palliative radiation generally takes time to achieve its effect. When radiation is planned near the EOL, up to 50% of patients do not receive all planned treatment.[12,44] In one series, 6 patients died during the course of radiation, 13 patients (21%) spent more than half of their last months receiving RT, and 43 (68%) were treated within 10 days of death.[12] In a national cohort of patients who died of incurable lung cancer, 10% received RT within 14 days of death and 16% of patients died during treatment.[44]

Given the time interval required for RT to achieve its palliative effect, patients with very short life expectancies are unlikely to benefit from RT. Accurate determinations and communication of survival estimates help patients avoid expensive treatment that may not alleviate their suffering or provide clinically significant benefits. Chapter 2 and Appendix B describe currently available predictive models that can help clinicians estimate life expectancy. Though these tools have limitations, they may be particularly helpful in selecting patients with very short survival for supportive care alone.

SUMMARY

PC for patients with advanced cancer requires multidisciplinary coordination. Prognostication and communication of accurate estimates of survival are essential to ensure the provision of appropriate care and avoid treatments that are unlikely to provide a benefit. Given the delay between radiation delivery and achievement of palliation, RT, especially prolonged courses of RT, should be avoided at the EOL. The shortest course of RT that will achieve the desired effect should be employed whenever possible to maximize patient comfort and convenience and minimize cost and toxicity.

RT palliates various local symptoms of advanced cancer including pain from bone metastasis or local tumor invasion, bleeding, obstruction, dyspnea, cough, and functional impairment due to brain metastasis or compression of the spinal cord or cauda equina. Short radiation regimens effectively palliate pain and other symptoms in most clinical scenarios. Side effects are typically self-limited and can be managed conservatively.

CLINICAL PEARLS

- RT plays a key role in the palliation of physical symptoms caused by advanced cancer and serves as an adjunct to systemic analgesics, chemotherapy, interventional procedures, and supportive care.
- The shortest course of palliative RT likely to have the desired effect should be employed. This maximizes patient comfort and convenience and minimizes cost and toxicity.
- Accurate determination and communication of survival estimates help patients set appropriate goals, avoid futile treatments, and choose supportive care or treatments that will be effective within their remaining lifetimes.

REFERENCES

1. Ferlay J, Soerjomataram I, Ervik M, et al. GLOBOCAN 2012 v1.0, Cancer Incidence and Mortality Worldwide: IARC Cancerbase No. 112013. http://globocan.iarc.fr. Accessed January 09, 2016.
2. Quill TE, Abernethy AP. Generalist plus specialist palliative care–creating a more sustainable model. *N Engl J Med*. March 28, 2013;368(13):1173-1175. PubMed PMID: 23465068.
3. Cohen SR, Mount BM, Tomas JJ, Mount LF. Existential well-being is an important determinant of quality of life. Evidence from the McGill Quality of Life Questionnaire. *Cancer*. February 1, 1996;77(3):576-586. PubMed PMID: 8630968.
4. Fisch MJ, Titzer ML, Kristeller JL, et al. Assessment of quality of life in outpatients with advanced cancer: the accuracy of clinician estimations and the relevance of spiritual well-being–a Hoosier Oncology Group Study. *J Clin Oncol*. July 15, 2003;21(14):2754-2759. PubMed PMID: 12860955.
5. Balboni TA, Paulk ME, Balboni MJ, et al. Provision of spiritual care to patients with advanced cancer: associations with medical care and quality of life near death. *J Clin Oncol*. January 20, 2010;28(3):445-452. PubMed PMID: 20008625. Pubmed Central PMCID: 2815706.
6. Balboni MJ, Sullivan A, Enzinger AC, et al. Nurse and physician barriers to spiritual care provision at the end of life. *J Pain Symptom Manage*. September 2014;48(3):400-410. PubMed PMID: 24480531. Pubmed Central PMCID: 4569089.
7. Borneman T, Ferrell B, Puchalski CM. Evaluation of the FICA Tool for Spiritual Assessment. *J Pain Symptom Manage*. 2010 Aug;40(2):163-173. Pubmed ID: 20619602.
8. Earle CC, Landrum MB, Souza JM, Neville BA, Weeks JC, Ayanian JZ. Aggressiveness of cancer care near the end of life: is it a quality-of-care issue? *J Clin Oncol*. August 10, 2008;26(23):3860-3866. PubMed PMID: 18688053. Pubmed Central PMCID: 2654813.
9. Earle CC, Park ER, Lai B, Weeks JC, Ayanian JZ, Block S. Identifying potential indicators of the quality of end-of-life cancer care from administrative data. *J Clin Oncol*. March 15, 2003;21(6):1133-1138. PubMed PMID: 12637481.
10. Hartsell WF, Desilvio M, Bruner DW, et al. Can physicians accurately predict survival time in patients with metastatic cancer? Analysis of RTOG 97-14. *J Palliat Med*. June 2008;11(5):723-728. PubMed PMID: 18588404. Epub 2008/07/01. eng.
11. Chow E, Harth T, Hruby G, Finkelstein J, Wu J, Danjoux C. How accurate are physicians' clinical predictions of survival and the available prognostic tools in estimating survival times in terminally ill cancer patients? A systematic review. *Clin Oncol (R Coll Radiol)*. 2001;13(3):209-218. PubMed PMID: 11527298.

12. Toole M, Lutz S, Johnstone PA. Radiation oncology quality: aggressiveness of cancer care near the end of life. *J Am Coll Radiol*. March 2012;9(3): 199-202. PubMed PMID: 22386167.

13. Hartsell WF, Scott, C, Bruner, DW et al. Phase III randomized trial of 8 Gy in 1 fraction vs. 30 Gy in 10 fractions for palliation of painful bone metastases: preliminary results of RTOG 97-14. *Int J Radiat Oncol Biol Phys*. 2003;57(suppl):124.

14. Johnstone C, Lutz ST. External beam radiotherapy and bone metastases. *Ann Palliat Med*. 2014;3(2):114-122.

15. Johnstone C, Lutz ST. The role of hypofractionated radiation in the management of non-osseous metastatic or uncontrolled local cancer. *Ann Palliat Med*. October, 2014;3(4):291-303. PubMed PMID: 25841909.

16. van den Hout WB, van der Linden YM, Steenland E, et al. Single- versus multiple-fraction radiotherapy in patients with painful bone metastases: cost–utility analysis based on a randomized trial. *J Natl Cancer Inst*. February 5, 2003;95(3):222-229. PubMed PMID: 12569144.

17. van der Linden YM, Steenland E, van Houwelingen HC, et al. Patients with a favourable prognosis are equally palliated with single and multiple fraction radiotherapy: results on survival in the Dutch Bone Metastasis Study. *Radiother Oncol*. 2006;78(3):245-253.

18. Macbeth FR, Bolger JJ, Hopwood P, et al. Randomized trial of palliative two-fraction versus more intensive 13-fraction radiotherapy for patients with inoperable non-small cell lung cancer and good performance status. Medical Research Council Lung Cancer Working Party. *Clin Oncol (R Coll Radiol)*. 1996;8(3):167-175. PubMed PMID: 8814371.

19. Simpson JR, Francis ME, Perez-Tamayo R, Marks RD, Rao DV. Palliative radiotherapy for inoperable carcinoma of the lung: final report of a RTOG multi-institutional trial. *Int J Radiat Oncol Biol Phys*. April, 1985;11(4): 751-758. PubMed PMID: 2579938.

20. Sundstrom S, Bremnes R, Aasebo U, et al. Hypofractionated palliative radiotherapy (17 Gy per two fractions) in advanced non-small-cell lung carcinoma is comparable to standard fractionation for symptom control and survival: a national phase III trial. *J Clin Oncol*. March 1, 2004;22(5):801-810. PubMed PMID: 14990635.

21. Duchesne GM, Bolger JJ, Griffiths GO, et al. A randomized trial of hypofractionated schedules of palliative radiotherapy in the management of bladder carcinoma: results of medical research council trial BA09. *Int J Radiat Oncol Biol Phys*. May 1, 2000;47(2):379-388. PubMed PMID: 10802363.

22. Chow E, Harris K, Fan G, Tsao M, Sze WM. Palliative radiotherapy trials for bone metastases: a systematic review. *J Clin Oncol*. 2007;25(11):1423-1436.

23. WHO. World Health Organization Pain Ladder 2010. http://www.who.int/cancer/palliative/painladder/en/. Accessed February 9, 2013.

24. Bhatt ML, Mohani BK, Kumar L, Chawla S, Sharma DN, Rath GK. Palliative treatment of advanced non small cell lung cancer with weekly fraction

radiotherapy. *Indian J Cancer*. December, 2000;37(4):148-152. PubMed PMID: 12018566.

25. Donato V, Zurlo A, Bonfili P, et al. Hypofractionated radiation therapy for inoperable advanced stage non-small cell lung cancer. *Tumori*. May–June, 1999;85(3):174-176. PubMed PMID: 10426127.

26. Lupattelli M, Maranzano E, Bellavita R, et al. Short-course palliative radiotherapy in non-small-cell lung cancer: results of a prospective study. *Am J Clin Oncol*. February, 2000;23(1):89-93. PubMed PMID: 10683087.

27. Rodrigues G, Macbeth F, Burmeister B, et al. Consensus statement on palliative lung radiotherapy: third international consensus workshop on palliative radiotherapy and symptom control. *Clin Lung Cancer*. January, 2012;13(1): 1-5. PubMed PMID: 21729656.

28. Stevens MJ, Begbie SD. Hypofractionated irradiation for inoperable non-small cell lung cancer. *Australas Radiol*. August, 1995;39(3):265-270. PubMed PMID: 7487763.

29. Vyas RK, Suryanarayana U, Dixit S, et al. Inoperable non-small cell lung cancer: palliative radiotherapy with two weekly fractions. *Indian J Chest Dis Allied Sci*. July–September, 1998;40(3):171-174. PubMed PMID: 9919836.

30. Kim DH, Lee JH, Ki YK, et al. Short-course palliative radiotherapy for uterine cervical cancer. *Radiat Oncol J*. December, 2013;31(4):216-221. PubMed PMID: 24501709. PubMed Central PMCID: 3912235.

31. Srinivasan V, Brown CH, Turner AG. A comparison of two radiotherapy regimens for the treatment of symptoms from advanced bladder cancer. *Clin Oncol (R Coll Radiol)*. 1994;6(1):11–13. PubMed PMID: 7513538.

32. Fairchild A, Barnes E, Ghosh S, et al. International patterns of practice in palliative radiotherapy for painful bone metastases: evidence-based practice? *Int J Radiat Oncol Biol Phys*. December 1, 2009;75(5):1501-1510. PubMed PMID: 19464820. Epub 2009/05/26. eng.

33. Lo SS, Lutz ST, Chang EL, et al. ACR appropriateness criteria® spinal bone metastases. *J Palliat Med*. January, 2013;16(1):9-19. PubMed PMID: 23167547. Epub 2012/11/22. eng.

34. Lutz ST, Berk L, Chang E, et al. Palliative radiotherapy for bone metastases: an ASTRO evidence-based guideline. *Int J Radiat Oncol Biol Phys*. March 15, 2011;79(4):965-976. PubMed PMID: 21277118. Epub 2011/02/01. eng.

35. Lutz ST, Lo SS, Chang EL, et al. ACR appropriateness criteria® non-spine bone metastases. *J Palliat Med*. May, 2012;15(5):521-526. PubMed PMID: 22536988. Epub 2012/04/28. eng.

36. NQF. #1822 External Beam Radiotherapy for Bone Metastasis. 2012.

37. ABIM. Choosing Wisely. 2012.

38. Ashworth A, Kong W, Chow E, Mackillop WJ. Fractionation of palliative radiation therapy for bone metastases in Ontario: do practice guidelines guide practice? *Int J Radiat Oncol Biol Phys*. January 1, 2016;94(1):31-39. PubMed PMID: 26454681.

39. Bekelman JE, Epstein AJ, Emanuel EJ. Single- vs multiple-fraction radiotherapy for bone metastases from prostate cancer. *JAMA*. October 9,

2013;310(14):1501-1502. PubMed PMID: 24104375. Pubmed Central PMCID: 4277868.

40. Ellsworth SG, Alcorn SR, Hales RK, McNutt TR, DeWeese TL, Smith TJ. Patterns of care among patients receiving radiation therapy for bone metastases at a large academic institution. *Int J Radiat Oncol Biol Phys*. August 1, 2014;89(5):1100-1105. PubMed PMID: 25035214. Pubmed Central PMCID: 4332799.

41. Olson RA, Tiwana MS, Barnes M, et al. Use of single- versus multiple-fraction palliative radiation therapy for bone metastases: population-based analysis of 16,898 courses in a Canadian province. *Int J Radiat Oncol Biol Phys*. August 1, 2014;89(5):1092-1099. PubMed PMID: 25035213.

42. Rutter CE, Yu JB, Wilson LD, Park HS. Assessment of national practice for palliative radiation therapy for bone metastases suggests marked underutilization of single-fraction regimens in the United States. *Int J Radiat Oncol Biol Phys*. March 1, 2015;91(3):548-555. PubMed PMID: 25542310.

43. Olson RA, Tiwana M, Barnes M, et al. Impact of using audit data to improve the evidence-based use of single-fraction radiation therapy for bone metastases in British Columbia. *Int J Radiat Oncol Biol Phys*. January 1, 2016;94(1):40-47. PubMed PMID: 26281828.

44. Kapadia NS, Mamet R, Zornosa C, Niland JC, D'Amico TA, Hayman JA. Radiation therapy at the end of life in patients with incurable nonsmall cell lung cancer. *Cancer*. September 1, 2012;118(17):4339-4345. PubMed PMID: 22252390.

2   Patient Selection and Life Expectancy Tools

Srinivas Raman, Nicholas Chiu, Na Zhang, and Edward Chow

INTRODUCTION

Life expectancy estimates for advanced cancer patients are necessary considerations in the fields of oncology and palliative care. While difficult to predict and uncomfortable to communicate, life expectancy estimates are important for a variety of clinical and personal reasons. In particular, accurate life expectancy estimates serve to: (a) guide appropriate clinical decisions, (b) direct planning of supportive services, (c) help patients and families plan end-of-life issues, (d) steer the allocation of resources, and (e) determine eligibility for hospice referrals or enrollment into clinical trials.

In terms of clinical decisions, the decision to treat, the modality of treatment, and the radiation dose schedule may all depend on survival prediction.[1] The decision between the use of supportive care alone versus radiation therapy (RT) in cases of complicated or uncomplicated bone metastases patients depends on life expectancy estimates.[2] Furthermore, a patient's treatment preferences, particularly in deliberating between life-extending therapies and palliative treatment, are influenced by the prognosis communicated to him or her.[3]

Survival estimates play an essential role in the planning of end-of-life issues and patients' and families' preparations for death. Steinhauser et al. conducted a cross-sectional, stratified random national survey to determine the factors considered important at the end of life by patients, families, physicians, and other providers.[4] An agreement was found across all groups on the need for symptom management, preparation for death, contemplation about one's life, being treated as a whole person, developing a relationship with medical care providers, and the usefulness of advance directives.[4] Moreover, in a study of patients' perspectives regarding quality end-of-life care, key domains of quality end-of-life care include the achievement of a sense of control and strengthened relationships with loved ones.[5] Addressing such factors in a limited time span requires accurate life expectancy estimates.

The allocation of resources and provision of cost-effective treatments require accurate survival prognosis.[6,7] Cost has become a key concern in reimbursement of expensive, high-technology procedures.[7] With shrinking resources and an aging population, the delivery of cancer treatment may require major changes as cancer patients of different ages and prognostic demographics compete for the same limited resources.[7] With regards to radiation oncology practices in particular, the use of single-fraction RT is more cost effective.[8]

Enrollment in hospice or a phase I clinical trial is often contingent on a patient's prognosis. To be considered for entry into phase I clinical trials, patients must typically have at least a 2- to 3-month estimated survival time, while that estimate is no more than 6 months for entry into a hospice program.[9] Temel et al. found that earlier referral to a hospice program leads to better management of patients' symptoms, stabilization of their conditions, and prolonged survival.[10] Given these factors, the importance of accurate survival estimates is evident, as they may aid in treatment decisions that could potentially boost quality of life and prolong survival.

This chapter on life expectancy and patient selection is written in recognition of the importance of accurate life expectancy estimates in the care of patients with advanced cancer. We describe some of the prognostic models currently available to help determine life expectancy and the limitations of those models. Furthermore, we discuss the changing landscape for prognostication in metastatic cancer, and elaborate on how survival estimates can affect clinical recommendations.

DESCRIPTIONS OF LIFE EXPECTANCY MODELS

Studies have found that a number of tumor factors, patient factors, and laboratory tests can be used to predict life expectancy in patients with advanced cancer.[11] Tumor factors are varied and broadly include primary tumor site and subtype, site(s) of metastases, and number of metastases. Metastatic breast cancer and prostate cancer are generally associated with a favorable prognosis compared to other cancers, but also this depends on the tumor subtype. For example, metastatic breast cancers with a triple negative biomarker profile have a more aggressive course and worse prognosis in comparison to metastatic breast cancers with a hormone receptor positive biomarker profile. This difference may be partially related to favorable biology, but the availability of therapeutic strategies that target the biology also contributes; for example, endocrine therapy for hormone positive breast cancer. The site(s) of metastatic disease is also an important factor. Patients with bone-only metastases generally have a more favorable prognosis than patients with involvement of visceral organs such as the liver and brain. Patients with a limited number of metastases can have prolonged survival and may benefit from more aggressive treatment.[12]

Patient factors usually include age, symptom burden, and performance status. Clinically significant symptoms predictive for survival include dyspnea, anorexia, nausea, xerostomia, confusion, mood, fatigue, and weight loss. Performance status is a measure of a patient's overall ability and functionality. The most commonly used metrics for performance status are Eastern Cooperative Oncology Group (ECOG) score, Karnofsky performance score (KPS), and palliative performance status (PPS). The KPS ranges from 0 to 100, where 100 is a perfect score with no functional impairment experienced by the patient and 0 is the worst score, signifying death. The PPS is similar to the KPS but also includes information about self-care, intake level, and consciousness level. The ECOG scale (also referred to as Zubrod or WHO scale) is similar to KPS/PPS but ranges from 0 to 5, where 0 represents an asymptomatic patient and 5 represents death. Performance status is predictive for survival. Multiple studies have found that a KPS less than 50 is consistently associated with a prognosis of less than 8 weeks.[13–17] Performance status is not solely predictive, particularly at higher KPS values or when KPS changes over time.[18] Laboratory tests, including lactate dehydrogenase (LDH), C-reactive protein (CRP), hemoglobin, white blood cell count/differential, and albumin level, have prognostic value when applied independently or in combination with other prognostic factors.[11]

To address the heterogeneity in patients with advanced cancers, numerous groups have proposed different multivariable life expectancy models using combinations of known tumor factors, patient factors, and laboratory tests. The most common indications for palliative RT include painful bone metastases, spinal cord compression, and brain metastases with the goals of symptom relief and/or local control. Local control is particularly important in brain metastases and spinal cord compression, as prompt treatment can mitigate, avoid, or delay neurologic compromise. Models developed for prognostication must reflect both the patient population and the goals of treatment. Accordingly, the focus of this section will be to introduce prognostic models developed specifically for patients who are seen in the setting of palliative RT. Appendix B contains prognostic models developed in other populations of patients that are particularly useful for predicting very short-term survival. Readers are also referred to an excellent review by Krishnan et al. for further information.[11]

Models Developed in the General Palliative RT Setting (Table 2.1)

A commonly used model for predicting life expectancy was developed by Chow et al. in patients with metastatic cancer attending an outpatient palliative RT clinic in Toronto, Canada.[19] The model was developed in a training dataset of 395 patients using a Cox's proportional hazards regression model.

From 16 prognostic factors, six prognostic factors were found to have a statistically significant impact on survival: primary cancer site, site of metastases, KPS, and fatigue, appetite, and shortness of breath scores from the modified Edmonton symptom assessment scale (ESAS). Both a survival prediction score (SPS) method and number of risk factors (NRF) method were used to predict survival. For the SPS method, each prognostic variable was assigned a weight based on the level of significance and a score from 0 to 32 was generated. The survival rates at different time points were determined for different SPS categories: ≤13, 14 to 19, and ≥20. The NRF method simply sums the total NRF present. Chow et al. validated the model on a temporal dataset in the same institution and an external dataset from a different institution.[20] Both the SPS and NRF discriminate survival in the three prognostic groups.

Chow et al. later simplified the model to include only three variables: (a) primary cancer site, (b) site of metastases, and (c) KPS.[20] Both the three and six variable models were found to predict survival similarly with no statistically significant difference in performance. The three-variable NRF model (non-breast primary cancer, metastases other than bone only, and KPS ≤60) is the simplest to use in clinic and performed similarly to the more complex models. It has been externally validated in an outpatient pain and palliative care clinic at Memorial Sloan Kettering Cancer Center[21] and in a palliative RT clinic in Norway.[22]

The TEACHH life expectancy model developed by Krishnan et al. identifies patients at different ends of the prognostic spectrum[23]; that is, patients having a life expectancy less than 3 months and greater than 1 year. The model was developed from a database of 862 patients with metastatic cancer who received palliative RT in Boston, United States. The median survival was 5.6 months. A Cox proportional hazards model and multivariate analysis identified factors predictive for a shorter life expectancy: T stands for primary tumor (lung and other vs. breast and prostate), E for ECOG performance status (2–4 vs. 0–1), A for older age (>60 vs. ≤60 years), C for prior palliative chemotherapy courses (≥2 vs. 0), H for hospitalizations within 3 months before palliative RT (0 vs. ≥1), and H for hepatic metastasis. Patients were divided into three groups with different median survivals: (a) group A (0–1 risk factors, overall survival [OS] = 19.9 months), (b) group B (2–4 risk factors, OS = 5 months), and (c) group C (5–6 risk factors, OS = 1.7 months).

Two models have been developed to predict those patients with a very poor prognosis, those with a life expectancy of less than 30 days.[24] Recursive partitioning analysis (RPA) was used to analyze 579 palliative RT courses at a single Norwegian institution. The median survival in the dataset was 6.3 months and the 30-day mortality was 9%. Factors predictive for 30-day mortality included primary lung or bladder cancer, ECOG PS 3–4, opioid use, steroid use, low hemoglobin, and progressive disease outside the RT volume.

(text continues on page 21)

TABLE 2.1 Life Expectancy Models, Developed in General Palliative RT Clinics

Author, Year	Patient Population	Median Survival	Description	Predicted Survival
Chow, 2002, 2008[19,20]	395 patients attending a palliative RT clinic at 2 Canadian institutions	19.4 wk	**NRF method (six variable)** A point assigned for each of the risk factors: ■ Non-breast cancer ■ Sites of metastases other than bone only ■ KPS ≤50 ■ ESAS Fatigue score 4–10 ■ ESAS Appetite score 8–10 ■ ESAS Shortness of breath score 1–10	Survival probabilities at 3, 6, and 12 mo: Group A (≤3): 85%, 72%, and 52% Group B (4): 68%, 47%, and 24% Group C (≥5): 46%, 24%, and 11%
			NRF method (three variable) A point assigned for each of the risk factors: ■ Non-breast cancer ■ Sites of metastases other than bone only ■ KPS ≤50	The median and 1-year survivals # Factors 0–1: 60 wk and 53% 2: 26 wk and 26% 3: 9 wk and 3%

(continued)

TABLE 2.1 Life Expectancy Models, Developed in General Palliative RT Clinics (*continued*)

Author, Year	Patient Population	Median Survival	Description	Predicted Survival
			SPS method Partial score in parenthesis assigned for risk factors in each category. ■ Primary cancer: Breast (0) Prostate (5) Lung (6) Other (7) ■ Site of metastasis: Bone only (0) Other (6) ■ KPS: >50 (0) ≤ 50 (6) ■ ESAS fatigue: 0 (0) 1–3 (0) 4–7 (4) 8–10 (5)	Survival probabilities at 3, 6, and 12 mo: Group A (≤13): 83%, 70%, and 51% Group B (14–19): 67%, 41%, and 20% Group C (≥20): 36%, 18%, and 4%

(*continued*)

TABLE 2.1 Life Expectancy Models, Developed in General Palliative RT Clinics (*continued*)

Author, Year	Patient Population	Median Survival	Description	Predicted Survival
			■ ESAS appetite: 0 (0) 1–3 (0) 4–7 (0) 8–10 (4) ■ ESAS dyspnea: 0 (0) 1–3 (2) 4–7 (4) 8–10 (4)	
Krishnan, 2014[23]	862 patients receiving palliative RT in a single U.S. institution	5.6 mo	One point assigned for presence of each of the risk factors: ■ Lung and other primary tumors (vs. breast and prostate) (**T**) ■ ECOG 2–4, (**E**) ■ Age >60 y, (**A**) ■ ≥2 prior palliative chemotherapy courses (**C**) ■ Presence of hepatic metastases (**H**) ■ ≥1 hospitalizations within 3 mo before palliative RT (**H**)	Median survival: Group A (0–1 points) = 19.9 mo Group B (2–4 points) = 5.0 mo Group C (5–6 points) = 1.7 mo

(*continued*)

TABLE 2.1 Life Expectancy Models, Developed in General Palliative RT Clinics (*continued*)

Author, Year	Patient Population	Median Survival	Description	Predicted Survival
Angelo, 2014[24]	579 palliative RT courses at a single Norwegian institution	6.3 mo	RPA with six-step decision tree ■ Lung/bladder primary ■ ECOG PS 3–4 ■ Opioid use ■ Low hemoglobin ■ Steroid use ■ Progressive disease outside RT volume	Patients meeting all six criteria had a 83% (training) and 84% (validation) death rate at 40 days
Spencer, 2015[25]	14,972 cases treated at a single U.K. institution	169 d	Male sex, nonbreast/nonprostate cancer, RT to multiple sites, and shorter fractionation were associated with higher rates of 30-d mortality	N/A

ECOG, Eastern Cooperative Oncology Group; ESAS, Edmonton symptom assessment scale; KPS, Karnofsky performance score; NRF, number of risk factors; RPA, recursive partitioning analysis; RT, radiation therapy; SPS, survival prediction score.

A larger population-based study of 14,972 cases treated at a single institution in the United Kingdom identified patients at risk of 30-day mortality after palliative RT.[25] Overall, the median survival was 5.6 months and the 30-day mortality was 12.3%. Factors predictive for 30-day mortality included sex, primary tumor, treatment site, and fractionation schedule.

Models Developed in Specific RT Settings (Table 2.2)

Models developed in patients with bone metastasis

Specific models for patients receiving RT to particular metastatic sites have also been developed for bone metastasis, spinal cord compression, and brain metastasis. van der Linden et al. developed a survival model from 342 patients in the Dutch Bone Metastasis study who received RT for painful Harrington Class I and II spinal metastases.[26] The median OS for all patients in the dataset was 7 months. A Cox proportional hazards model and multivariate analysis identified the major predictors for survival: KPS (10–40, 50–70, 80–100), primary tumor site (breast, prostate, lung), and presence of visceral metastases. A score was assigned to each category and the final classification system included three groups. Group A had a median OS of 3 months, Group B had a median OS of 9 months, and Group C had a median OS of 18.7 months. The patients in Group C had the most favorable prognostic features: primary breast cancer, good performance status, and absence of visceral metastasis. Westhoff et al. developed a prognostic model from the larger cohort of 1,157 patients enrolled in the Dutch Bone Metastasis study.[27] The median survival for the patients in the dataset was 30 weeks. Univariate and multivariate Cox proportional hazard models with backward selection were used to select and combine the variables most predictive for survival. The best predictive model had a C-statistic of 0.72 and included sex, primary cancer site (breast, prostate, lung, other), presence of visceral metastases, KPS (90–100, 70–80, 20–60), general health rating on a visual analog scale (VAS-gh 67–100, 34–66, 0–33) and valuation of life on a verbal rating scale (VRS-vl 1–3, 4, 5–7). A simplified model with a C-statistic of 0.71 identified KPS and primary cancer site as prognostic variables. Median survival and survival rates at 3, 6, 9, 12, and 18 months were reported for each combination. External validation of the model was performed in a separate dataset of 934 patients at a single Dutch Institution with a C-statistic of 0.72 and a similar calibration plot.

Chow et al. developed a survival prediction model from patients with a KPS ≥50 undergoing reirradiation for bone metastases in the SC-20 trial.[28] The training and model validation datasets included 460 and 351 patients, respectively. A Cox regression model using backward selection was used to select statistically significant variables; only KPS and primary tumor site were found to be predictive for survival. Partial scores were assigned to KPS (90–100,

(text continues on page 25)

TABLE 2.2 Life Expectancy Models, Developed Using Patients With Specific RT Indications

Author, Year	Patient Population	Median Survival	Description	Predicted Survival
van der Linden, 2005[26]	342 patients receiving RT to spine in Dutch Bone Metastases study	7 mo	Points in parentheses assigned for risk factors in each category: ■ KPS: 80–100 (2) 50–70 (1) 10–40 (0) ■ Primary tumor site: Breast (3) Prostate (2) Lung (1) Other (0) ■ Visceral metastases: No (0) Yes (1)	Median survival: Group A (0–3 points) = 3.0 mo Group B (4–5 points) = 9.0 mo Group C (6 points) = 18.7 mo
Westhoff, 2014[27]	1,157 patients enrolled in Dutch Bone Metastases study	30 wk	Predictive factors (sex, primary tumor, visceral metastases, KPS, patient reported general health on a visual analogue scale and valuation of life on a VRS) were associated with survival, details of model not presented.	Readers are directed to the original publication for a table of observed survivals for different primary tumors and KPS.

(continued)

TABLE 2.2 Life Expectancy Models, Developed Using Patients With Specific RT Indications (*continued*)

Author, Year	Patient Population	Median Survival	Description	Predicted Survival
Chow, 2015[28]	460 patients (training) and 351 patients (testing) undergoing reirradiation for bone metastases in the SC-20 trial	9.3–9.7 mo	**SPS:** Points in parentheses assigned for risk factors in each category. ■ KPS: 90–100 (0) 70–80 (1) 50–60 (2) ■ Primary tumor: Breast (0) Prostate (1.3) Other (2.6) Lung (3)	Survival probabilities at 3, 6, and 12 mo in testing set: Group A (≤2): 94%, 85%, and 65% Group B (2.1–3.6): 85%, 68%, and 48% Group C (>3.6): 64%, 43%, and 20%
Rades, 2008[29]	1,852 patients treated with RT for spinal cord compression at multiple institutions	Unknown	Points in parentheses are assigned for risk factors in each category: ■ Primary tumor: Breast (8) Prostate (7)	Survival probabilities at 6 mo Group A (20–25 points) = 4% Group B (26–30 points) = 11% Group C (31–35 points) = 48% Group D (36–40 points) = 87% Group E (41–45 points) = 99%

(*continued*)

TABLE 2.2 Life Expectancy Models, Developed Using Patients With Specific RT Indications (*continued*)

Author, Year	Patient Population	Median Survival	Description	Predicted Survival
			Myeloma/lymphoma (9)	
			Lung (3)	
			Others (4)	
			■ Other bone metastases at RT:	
			Yes (5)	
			No (7)	
			■ Visceral metastases at RT:	
			Yes (2)	
			No (8)	
			■ Interval from diagnosis to MSCC:	
			≤15 mo (4)	
			>15 mo (7)	
			■ Ambulatory status before RT:	
			Ambulatory (7)	
			Nonambulatory (3)	
			■ Time to develop motor deficits before RT:	
			1–7 d (3)	
			8–14 d (6)	
			>14 d (8)	

KPS, Karnofsky performance score; MSCC, malignant spinal cord compression; RT, radiation therapy; SPS, survival prediction score; VRS, verbal rating scale.

70–80, 50–60) and primary tumor site (breast, prostate, lung). An SPS ranging from 0 to 5 was generated where the 1/3 and 2/3 percentile scores were 2 and 3.6, respectively. In the testing dataset, the median survival for the group with the best prognosis was not reached. In the other two groups, the median survivals were 11.3 and 5.2 months. The 3-, 6-, and 12-month survival rates for the worst group were 64.4%, 43.0%, and 19.7%, respectively.

Malignant spinal cord compression (MSCC) is caused by displacement or compression of the spinal cord by tumor and is described in detail in Chapter 4. MSCC can be associated with significant morbidity despite aggressive and emergent intervention; the prognosis for MSCC is thought to differ from uncomplicated spinal and bone metastases. A scoring system was developed using six factors found to be significant on a multivariate analysis of 1,852 patients undergoing RT for MSCC at multiple international institutions: tumor type, interval between cancer diagnosis and development of MSCC, presence of other sites of disease, ambulatory status, and duration of motor deficits.[29] Each factor was assigned a prognostic score. The summed scores were then divided into five categories with 6-month survival rates of 4%, 11%, 48%, 87%, and 99%. In the two categories with the highest 6-month survival, long-course RT, defined as 10 to 20 fractions delivered over 2 to 4 weeks, was associated with a statistically significant improvement in survival. This prognostic model was validated by a separate dataset of 439 patients with similar 6-month survival rates.[30] The model was simplified with different prognostic score cut-offs and associated 6-month survivals of 14%, 56%, and 80%.[30]

Models Developed in Patients With Brain Metastasis

With an incidence of 10% to 20% in patients with cancer,[31] brain metastases are a common indication for palliative RT. Prognostication represents a unique challenge in the treatment of patients with brain metastasis since only 30% to 50% of patients will die from their brain metastasis. Predictive models need to account for successful control of both intracranial and extracranial disease since both are closely tied to prognosis. Gaspar et al. developed the RPA using data from 1,200 patients from three Radiation Therapy Oncology Group (RTOG) trials: 79-16, 85-28, and 89-05. All patients received whole brain RT (WBRT), with a subset of patients in RTOG 85-28 receiving a boost dose.[32] Based on the analysis of 18 pretreatment and three treatment-related variables, three RPA categories were developed (Table 2.3).

The RPA model was independently validated in a dataset of 432 patients from RTOG 91-04.[33] This tool was later validated in a separate population not included in the RTOG trials, patients with small-cell lung cancer.[34] A potential criticism of this tool is that it was developed in patients who presented with symptomatic brain metastases in an era that predated routine magnetic

TABLE 2.3 RPA Classification and Median Survival by Class

		Median Survival	
RPA Class	**Factors**	**Initial Dataset**	**Validation Dataset**
Class 1	Age <65 KPS ≥70 Controlled primary tumor No extracranial disease	7.1 mo	6.2 mo
Class 2	All other patients	4.2 mo	3.8 mo
Class 3	KPS <70	2.3 mo	n/a

KPS, Karnofsky performance score; RPA, recursive partitioning analysis.

resonance imaging (MRI); today, many patients present with asymptomatic brain metastases incidentally found on MRI.

To incorporate the number of brain metastases, which is also a prognostic factor, Sperduto et al. developed the graded prognostic assessment (GPA) in a database of 1,960 patients from four RTOG trials.[35] A score of 0, 0.5, or 1 was assigned to the following categories: age, KPS, number of brain metastases, and presence of extracranial metastases. The median survival times for the four GPA categories were 2.6, 3.8, 6.9, and 11.0 months. Due to heterogeneity in the primary tumor sites and implications on prognosis, Sperduto et al. also subsequently developed a diagnosis-specific GPA (DS-GPA). From a database of 3,940 patients, a multivariate analysis identified the most prognostic variables for each primary tumor site and a GPA score was assigned to each variable.[36] Median survival resulting from disease-specific GPA was reported for patients with lung cancer, melanoma, breast cancer, renal cell carcinoma, and gastrointestinal cancers (Table 2.4).

The RPA, GPA, and DS-GPA are the most commonly used tools for predicting life expectancy in patients with brain metastases and the majority of current clinical trials in brain metastases still use these indices as stratification factors. However, numerous other life expectancy tools have also been developed for use in brain metastases, including the Rotterdam system,[37] the score index of radiosurgery,[38] the basic score for brain metastases,[39] the Golden grading system,[40] and the two classification systems developed by Rades et al.[41,42] Readers are directed to an excellent systematic review by Rodrigues et al. for further description and performance of the various prognostic indices in patients with brain metastasis.[43]

INACCURACY OF LIFE EXPECTANCY ESTIMATES AND LIMITATIONS OF LIFE EXPECTANCY MODELS

Inaccurate life expectancy estimates by physicians have been well documented in the literature.[3,6,44–46] Survival predictions by physicians are often

TABLE 2.4 Prognostic Factors From the DS-RPA

Specific Cancer Type	Prognostic Factors
Lung cancer	Age
	KPS
	Extracranial metastases
	Number of brain metastasis
Melanoma	KPS
	Number of brain metastasis
Breast cancer	Age
	KPS
	Subtype
Renal cell carcinoma	KPS
	Number of brain metastasis
Gastrointestinal cancers	KPS

KPS, Karnofsky performance score.

overly optimistic,[1,44,46] although Janisch et al. found that they can be overly pessimistic as well.[45] Six radiation oncologists provided survival estimates for 739 patients in a study by Chow et al.[1] Physicians overestimated survival by more than 3 months. Similarly, Chistakis et al. found that 63% of physician estimates were overly optimistic, while 17% were overly pessimistic.[46] The results of such studies underscore the inaccuracy of clinical life expectancy estimates on the part of physicians.

The issue of inaccurate estimates is not trivial, as overly optimistic beliefs may prevent earlier palliative care.[47] This can have direct consequences on survival, as Temel et al.'s randomized controlled trial (RCT) demonstrated that metastatic non–small-cell lung cancer (NSCLC) patients treated with early palliative care lived longer than their counterparts treated with standard oncologic care alone.[10] Furthermore, a study of 917 adults by Weeks et al. found that even when physician estimates were less optimistic, many patients overestimated their odds of surviving by at least 6 months.[3] These patients were two times more likely to favor life-extending therapy rather than palliative care when compared with those who indicated that they had at least a 10% chance of death within 6 months. Importantly, after controlling for other prognostic factors, 6-month survival was no better for those patients who underwent aggressive treatment.

The negative consequences associated with patient misinformation about true survival prognosis are evident. Nevertheless, physicians often do not communicate such information to their patients.[9,48] They did not communicate a survival estimate (22%) or communicated a different estimate than they

formulated (40%) for the majority of patients. They communicated the estimate they formulated only 37% of the time. Lamont et al. reasoned that physicians might be subject to an optimism bias, causing them to unconsciously
make errors in estimating patients' prognoses. They also raised the possibility that physicians consciously communicate erroneous survival estimates
to patients due to the belief that an unfavorable prognosis could adversely
affect a patient's quality of life and possibly survival. More often, adverse
consequences such as dying in the hospital or seeking overly aggressive care
results from overly optimistic survival estimates. Thus, the importance of providing truthful and accurate estimates about a patient's survival cannot be
overemphasized.[48]

Prognostic models for predicting survival generally produce more accurate estimates of life expectancy than clinical estimates. Due to continuously
evolving treatments, these models may be incomplete or become outdated.
For example in the last 5 years, landmark studies in patients with metastatic
prostate cancer demonstrated survival advantages with three new systemic
therapies: abiraterone,[49,50] enzalutamide,[51,52] and radium-223.[53] Particularly
relevant to the field of palliative radiation oncology, there is also accruing evidence that the choice of therapy for brain metastases may affect survival[54] and
current prognostic indexes do not take this factor into account. Evidence also
suggests that in very advanced stages of cancer, treatments do not significantly
extend the quantity of life. In a systemic review by Salpeter et al., "terminal"
presentations of various cancers with an associated survival of 6 months or
less were reviewed.[55] In this terminal phase, treatment of the underlying cancer
did not prolong survival.

The most likely explanation for this apparent discrepancy is patient selection. In clinical trials, the inclusion/exclusion criterion is determined so that
if the experimental therapy is beneficial, the patient population will live long
enough to show the hypothesized difference. Therefore, although treatments
must be taken into consideration for a prognostic model to be accurate, the
effects of the interventions may not be as robust in a general population.

ADVANCED PREDICTION MODELS AND INTEGRATION OF BIOMARKERS

The past two decades have seen remarkable advances in understanding
the molecular biology of cancer and how it affects malignant behavior and
response to systemic therapy. This information is commonly used in the
medical oncology setting for selecting the optimal chemotherapeutic strategy.
However, much of this information is not routinely used to guide decision
making in RT.

The discovery of epidermal growth factor receptor (EGFR) mutation and
anaplastic lymphoma kinase (ALK) fusion in NSCLC has demonstrated the

heterogeneity in the clinical outcomes of patients with metastatic NSCLC when treated with targeted therapy. Patients with EGFR mutation have better survival outcomes and increased responsiveness to targeted therapies in comparison to patients with wild type lung cancers.[56] Similarly in metastatic breast cancer, patients with hormone receptor positivity have a significantly more favorable prognosis than those with hormone receptor negative or triple negative tumors. Despite having a significant burden of disease or poor prognostic features, patients with EGFR-mutated NSCLC and hormone receptor-positive breast cancer can have a good response to EGFR-targeted therapy and endocrine therapy, respectively, with a favorable toxicity profile and prolonged survival.

As the number of known biomarkers and prognostic tools increase, efforts must be made to integrate these tools in the RT clinic. There must be a balance between the use of the best and most up-to-date prognostic models without increasing the complexity of the model such that it becomes cumbersome for routine use. Machine learning techniques[57] present promising methods to incorporate advanced prediction through well designed, intuitive user interfaces in the clinic.

HOW DOES LIFE EXPECTANCY AFFECT PATIENT SELECTION AND CLINICAL RECOMMENDATIONS FOR PALLIATIVE RT?

Bone Metastases

For uncomplicated, painful bone metastases, there is evidence to suggest that most patients benefit from palliative RT and therefore treatment should be offered to all patients. Several studies demonstrate that elderly patients benefit from RT at the same rate as younger patients.[58,59] Two series evaluated pain response in patients who died within 3 months of palliative RT for bone metastasis.[60,61] Between 45% and 70% of patients report decreased pain during their remaining lives. In the Dutch Bone Metastases Study cohort, there was no difference in the efficacy between single-fraction and multiple-fraction treatment.[62] As will be discussed in Chapter 3, there are multiple RCTs and a large meta-analysis that show the equivalence of single-fraction and multiple-fraction radiation treatment in the treatment of uncomplicated bone metastasis and in retreatment of painful bone lesions. Since single-fraction radiation is equally effective at palliating pain, it should be the preferred regimen in all patients, but especially for those within 3 months of death.

There is little evidence to suggest that life expectancy should dramatically affect patient selection and clinical recommendations for uncomplicated bone metastases. Since maximal pain relief typically takes 3 to 5 weeks, those patients with a life expectancy less than 1 month probably will not benefit from this treatment, though some patients can experience relief in as little as 24 to 48 hours. If treatment is attempted, it should be with a single fraction of radiation.

Malignant Spinal Cord Compression

In MSCC, there is retrospective evidence that suggests that patient selection and life expectancy should guide recommendations for RT. Rades et al. observed that long course (10–20 fractions) RT was associated with better local control than short course (1–5 fractions) RT and there was a trend toward better OS favoring long-course RT.[63,64] In developing their model for prognostication in MSCC, Rades et al. observed that long-course RT was only predictive for OS in those patients with favorable prognosis, defined as a score greater than 36 points in their model.[29]

Maranzano et al. randomized 327 patients with a short life expectancy (≤6 months) to one of two short course RT schedules for management of SCC,[65] either 8 Gy in 1 fraction or 2 fractions (16 Gy). Both treatment schedules were equally effective with no observed difference in response rates or median survival. The median survival was 4 months with a median follow-up of 31 months; thus, not all patients had a short survival.

Rades et al. performed a retrospective, matched-pair analysis comparing a radiation dose of 37.5 Gy in 15 fractions or 40 Gy in 20 fractions with 30 Gy in 10 fractions for MSCC in patients with a favorable prognosis, defined as a score of ≥36 on their prognostic indexes.[66] The 191 patients were selected from each category. Local control rates at 2 years in the 30- and 36 Gy arm were 71% and 92%, respectively. Progression free and OSs were higher in the low-dose and high-dose arm. Escalating the radiation dose beyond 30 Gy may be beneficial in selected patients but selection bias inherent in retrospective analyses may be present.

In patients with a short life expectancy, longer courses of RT with higher doses do not provide any significant benefit. For uncomplicated bone metastasis, there is no benefit to longer courses of radiation when compared with single-fraction regimens. In patients with MSCC, those with a favorable prognosis may benefit from long-course RT, as they may survive long enough to realize the benefit in local control (see Chapter 4 for additional detail).

Brain Metastasis

The decisions surrounding optimal management of patients with multiple or unresectable brain metastases are evolving and there are many factors that help clinicians choose between WBRT and stereotactic radiosurgery (SRS). This topic is discussed extensively in Chapter 6. There is a growing trend toward SRS alone, if possible, to prevent the undesirable effect of neurocognitive decline from WBRT.[67] WBRT may be appropriate for patients with numerous metastases, large metastases, uncontrolled systemic disease, and/or a poor prognosis.[31]

Patients with a very poor prognosis or short life expectancy may not benefit from WBRT. Windsor et al. reviewed a cohort of 3,459 patients who underwent WBRT at three institutions between 1991 and 2007.[68] Seventeen percent of treated patients died within 6 weeks of radiation. Older age, a short interval between primary cancer diagnosis and WBRT, and repeat WBRT all predicted increased mortality within 6 weeks. Although WBRT is usually well tolerated, acute toxicities, including headaches, fatigue, nausea/vomiting, radiation dermatitis, and alopecia, can reduce quality of life. Optimal supportive care alone may be preferable in these patients. The QUARTZ trial is an ongoing randomized, noninferiority phase III study that compares optimal supportive care plus WBRT versus optimal supportive care alone for patients with NSCLC and inoperable brain metastases. A preliminary analysis of 538 patients[69] suggested that there was no difference in survival between the WBRT arm (65 days) and the supportive care alone arm (57 days). The poor median survivals in both arms suggest that the enrolled patients had a poor baseline prognosis and may represent enrollment bias. Further research is required to determine which patients may not benefit from the addition of WBRT for brain metastases.

Oligometastases

Although there are varying definitions for oligometastases, one such description is that it represents a subset of metastatic disease where the burden of disease is limited and there exists potential for long-term disease eradication or control with local, radical treatment of the metastatic lesions. Patients with oligometastatic disease who most likely benefit from stereotactic body RT (SBRT) have a long disease free survival, breast histology, 1 to 3 metastases, small metastases, and receive higher doses of radiation.[12] There is significant overlap between these characteristics and variables predictive for a favorable prognosis in the previously described life expectancy models. Therefore, patients with oligometastatic disease and a favorable life expectancy should be considered for more radical treatment. Since there is a tendency to overestimate prognoses, objective criteria and models (described previously), should be used to help determine which patients may potentially benefit from more aggressive treatment.

SUMMARY

Accurate prognostication in patients with advanced cancer is extremely important in the palliative RT setting. It impacts treatment recommendations, decisions to enroll in a clinical trial, and the organization of appropriate support services. It can also guide patient expectations and allow them to make necessary arrangements and may impact their desire for aggressive end-of-life care. Furthermore, it can also help optimize resource allocation from a health care system perspective.

Various prognostication models that were developed in a variety of clinical contexts, ranging from a general outpatient palliative RT clinic to patients treated on specific clinical trials for spinal cord compression, and bone and brain metastases, were described along with their limitations. These models can help select patients for particular palliative radiation treatments and fractionation regimens and offer insight as to when supportive care alone may be best. Some of these models will likely change and adapt as our understanding of cancer and cancer biomarkers evolves.

CLINICAL PEARLS

- Accurate prognostication and communication of life expectancy estimates in patients with advanced cancer is extremely important in the palliative RT setting. This helps guide appropriate clinical decisions and avoid futile or overly aggressive treatment, helps patients and families plan end-of-life issues, helps steer the allocation of resources, and helps determine eligibility for hospice referrals or enrollment into clinical trials.
- Physicians generally overestimate life expectancy by 3 months or more. Prognostic models for predicting survival are generally more accurate than clinical estimates.
- The NRF and TEACHH predictive models are relatively simple prognostic models that are generalizable to all patients seen in an RT clinic.
- The best use of life expectancy estimates may be in determining which patients may not live long enough to benefit from a particular therapeutic intervention.

SELF-ASSESSMENT

Questions

1. Which tool would you use to estimate the life expectancy of a 65-year-old woman newly diagnosed with lung cancer metastatic to the liver and bone who has a KPS of 90 (ECOG 0)?
   A. NRF-3
   B. TEACHH
   C. DS-GPA

2. What is the median life expectancy in months of a 65-year-old woman newly diagnosed with lung cancer metastatic to the liver and bone who has a KPS of 90 (ECOG 1)?
   A. 1 to 2 months
   B. 5 to 6 months
   C. 9 to 10 months
   D. >12 months

3. If this patient had brain metastasis, what additional information would you need to determine her median survival?
   A. Symptoms from brain metastasis
   B. Size of the brain metastasis
   C. Number of brain metastases
   D. Location of brain metastasis

4. Which patient may not live long enough to see the benefit of WBRT and may best be treated with dexamethasone and supportive care?

Patient	Age/Gender	Tumor Type	KPS (ECOG)	Extent of Disease
A	80 F	Breast	80 (1)	Bone, brain
B	66 F	Breast	50 (3)	Bone, brain
C	80 M	Lung	70 (1)	Bone, brain
D	66 M	Lung	50 (3)	Brain, liver

Answers

1. Answer A. Though both the NRF-3 and TEACHH models were developed for general populations, the best tool in this scenario would be to use the NRF-3 as all of the factors are detailed in the case history. The DS-GPA is only applicable to patients with brain metastasis.

2. Answer B. With the NRF-3 model, this patient gets one point for a lung primary and one for liver metastases (nonbone site). Her KPS is greater than 60, so she does not get points for this. With a total of two points, her median survival is 26 weeks and 1-year OS is 26%. If you knew that she had no prior chemotherapy and no prior hospitalizations, you could use the TEACHH tool. She would have a score of 3, with one point for her age greater than 60, one for the presence of hepatic metastasis, and one for lung cancer tumor type. With this score, she would have a median survival of 20 weeks.

3. Answer C. In a patient with brain metastasis, to use the lung specific GPA, additional prognostic factors are the number of brain metastases and the presence or absence of extracranial disease. Her age and KPS are already known.

4. Answer D. Factors predictive of a high 30-day mortality include KPS ≤50 (ECOG 3–4), bladder or lung cancer, use of opioids or steroids, a low hemoglobin, and progressive disease outside the radiation field. Performance status is a stronger predictor of survival than age.

REFERENCES

1. Chow E, Davis L, Panzarella T, et al. Accuracy of survival prediction by palliative radiation oncologists. *Int J Radiat Oncol Biol Phys*. 2005;61(3):870-873.
2. Chiu N, Chiu L, Lutz S, et al. Incorporation of life expectancy estimates in the treatment of palliative care patients receiving radiotherapy: treatment approaches in light of incomplete prognostic models. *Ann Palliat Med*. 2015;4(3):162-168.
3. Weeks JC, Cook EF, O'Day SJ, et al. Relationship between cancer patients' predictions of prognosis and their treatment preferences. *JAMA*. 1998;279(21):1709-1714.
4. Steinhauser KE, Christakis NA, Clipp EC, et al. Factors considered important at the end of life by patients, family, physicians, and other care providers. *JAMA*. 2000;284(19):2476-2482.
5. Singer PA, Martin DK, Kelner M. Quality end-of-life care: patients' perspectives. *JAMA*. 1999;281(2):163-168.
6. Maher E. How long have I got doctor? *Eur J Cancer*. 1994;30(3):283-284.
7. Smith TJ, Hillner BE, Desch CE. Efficacy and cost-effectiveness of cancer treatment: rational allocation of resources based on decision analysis. *J Natl Cancer Inst*. 1993;85(18):1460-1474.
8. van der Linden YM, Steenland E, van Houwelingen HC, et al. Patients with a favourable prognosis are equally palliated with single and multiple fraction radiotherapy: results on survival in the Dutch Bone Metastasis Study. *Radiother Oncol*. 2006;78(3):245-253.
9. Lamont EB, Christakis NA. Some elements of prognosis in terminal cancer. *Oncology (Williston Park, NY)*. 1999;13(8):1165-1170; discussion 72-74, 79-80.
10. Temel JS, Greer JA, Muzikansky A, et al. Early palliative care for patients with metastatic non–small-cell lung cancer. *N Engl J Med*. 2010;363(8):733-742.
11. Krishnan M, Temel JS, Wright AA, et al. Predicting life expectancy in patients with advanced incurable cancer: a review. *J Support Oncol*. 2013;11(2):68-74.
12. Tree AC, Khoo VS, Eeles RA, et al. Stereotactic body radiotherapy for oligometastases. *Lancet Oncol*. 2013;14(1):e28-e37.
13. Evans C, Mccarthy M. Prognostic uncertainty in terminal care: can the Karnofsky index help? *Lancet*. 1985;325(8439):1204-1206.

14. Maltoni M, Nanni O, Derni S, et al. Clinical prediction of survival is more accurate than the Karnofsky performance status in estimating life span of terminally ill cancer patients. *Eur J Cancer*. 1994;30(6):764-766.

15. Maltoni M, Pirovano M, Scarpi E, et al. Prediction of survival of patients terminally III with cancer. Results of an Italian prospective multicentric study. *Cancer*. 1995;75(10):2613-2622.

16. Reuben DB, Mor V, Hiris J. Clinical symptoms and length of survival in patients with terminal cancer. *Arch Intern Med*. 1988;148(7):1586-1591.

17. Llobera J, Esteva M, Rifa J, et al. Terminal cancer: duration and prediction of survival time. *Eur J Cancer*. 2000;36(16):2036-2043.

18. Yates JW, Chalmer B, McKegney FP. Evaluation of patients with advanced cancer using the Karnofsky performance status. *Cancer*. 1980;45(8):2220-2224.

19. Chow E, Fung K, Panzarella T, et al. A predictive model for survival in metastatic cancer patients attending an outpatient palliative radiotherapy clinic. *Int J Radiat Oncol Biol Phys*. 2002;53(5):1291-1302.

20. Chow E, Abdolell M, Panzarella T, et al. Predictive model for survival in patients with advanced cancer. *J Clin Oncol*. 2008;26(36):5863-5869.

21. Glare P, Shariff I, Thaler HT. External validation of the number of risk factors score in a palliative care outpatient clinic at a comprehensive cancer center. *J Palliat Med*. 2014;17(7):797-802.

22. Angelo K, Dalhaug A, Pawinski A, et al. Survival prediction score: a simple but age-dependent method predicting prognosis in patients undergoing palliative radiotherapy. *ISRN Oncol*. 2014;2014.

23. Krishnan MS, Epstein-Peterson Z, Chen YH, et al. Predicting life expectancy in patients with metastatic cancer receiving palliative radiotherapy: the TEACHH model. *Cancer*. 2014;120(1):134-141.

24. Angelo K, Norum J, Dalhaug A, et al. Development and validation of a model predicting short survival (death within 30 days) after palliative radiotherapy. *Anticancer Res*. 2014;34(2):877-885.

25. Spencer K, Morris E, Dugdale E, et al. 30 day mortality in adult palliative radiotherapy—A retrospective population based study of 14,972 treatment episodes. *Radiother Oncol*. 2015;115(2):264-271.

26. van der Linden YM, Dijkstra SP, Vonk EJ, et al. Prediction of survival in patients with metastases in the spinal column. *Cancer*. 2005;103(2):320-328.

27. Westhoff PG, de Graeff A, Monninkhof EM, et al. An easy tool to predict survival in patients receiving radiation therapy for painful bone metastases. *Int J Radiat Oncol Biol Phys*. 2014;90(4):739-747.

28. Chow E, Ding K, Parulekar WR, et al. Predictive model for survival in patients having repeat radiation treatment for painful bone metastases. *Radiother Oncol*. 2016;118(3):547-551.

29. Rades D, Dunst J, Schild SE. The first score predicting overall survival in patients with metastatic spinal cord compression. *Cancer*. 2008;112(1):157-161.

30. Rades D, Douglas S, Veninga T, et al. Validation and simplification of a score predicting survival in patients irradiated for metastatic spinal cord compression. *Cancer*. 2010;116(15):3670-3673.

31. Lin X, DeAngelis LM. Treatment of brain metastases. *J Clin Oncol*. 2015;33(30):3475-3484.

32. Gaspar L, Scott C, Rotman M, et al. Recursive partitioning analysis (RPA) of prognostic factors in three Radiation Therapy Oncology Group (RTOG) brain metastases trials. *Int J Radiat Oncol Biol Phys*. 1997;37(4):745-751.

33. Gaspar LE, Scott C, Murray K, Curran W. Validation of the RTOG recursive partitioning analysis (RPA) classification for brain metastases. *Int J Radiat Oncol Biol Phys*. 2000;47(4):1001-1006.

34. Videtic GM, Adelstein DJ, Mekhail TM, et al. Validation of the RTOG recursive partitioning analysis (RPA) classification for small-cell lung cancer–only brain metastases. *Int J Radiat Oncol Biol Phys*. 2007;67(1):240-243.

35. Sperduto PW, Berkey B, Gaspar LE, et al. A new prognostic index and comparison to three other indices for patients with brain metastases: an analysis of 1,960 patients in the RTOG database. *Int J Radiat Oncol Biol Phys*. 2008;70(2):510-514.

36. Sperduto PW, Kased N, Roberge D, et al. Summary report on the graded prognostic assessment: an accurate and facile diagnosis-specific tool to estimate survival for patients with brain metastases. *J Clin Oncol*. 2012;30(4):419-425. PubMed PMID: 22203767. Pubmed Central PMCID: 3269967.

37. Lagerwaard F, Levendag P, Nowak PC, et al. Identification of prognostic factors in patients with brain metastases: a review of 1292 patients. *Int J Radiat Oncol Biol Phys*. 1999;43(4):795-803.

38. Weltman E, Salvajoli JV, Brandt RA, et al. Radiosurgery for brain metastases: a score index for predicting prognosis. *Int J Radiat Oncol Biol Phys*. 2000;46(5):1155-1161.

39. Lorenzoni J, Devriendt D, Massager N, et al. Radiosurgery for treatment of brain metastases: estimation of patient eligibility using three stratification systems. *Int J Radiat Oncol Biol Phys*. 2004;60(1):218-224.

40. Golden DW, Lamborn KR, McDermott MW, et al. Prognostic factors and grading systems for overall survival in patients treated with radiosurgery for brain metastases: variation by primary site. *J Neurosurg*. 2008;109:77–86.

41. Rades D, Dunst J, Schild SE. A new scoring system to predicting the survival of patients treated with whole-brain radiotherapy for brain metastases. *Strahlenther Onkol*. 2008;184(5):251-255.

42. Rades D, Dziggel L, Haatanen T, et al. Scoring systems to estimate intracerebral control and survival rates of patients irradiated for brain metastases. *Int J Radiat Oncol Biol Phys*. 2011;80(4):1122-1127.

43. Rodrigues G, Bauman G, Palma D, et al. Systematic review of brain metastases prognostic indices. *Pract Radiat Oncol*. 2013;3(2):101-106.

44. Chow E, Harth T, Hruby G, et al. How accurate are physicians' clinical predictions of survival and the available prognostic tools in estimating survival

times in terminally iII cancer patients? A systematic review. *Clin Oncol (R Coll Radiol)*. 2001;13(3):209-218.

45. Janisch L, Mick R, Schilsky RL, et al. Prognostic factors for survival in patients treated in phase I clinical trials. *Cancer*. 1994;74(7):1965-1973.

46. Christakis NA, Smith JL, Parkes CM, Lamont EB. Extent and determinants of error in doctors' prognoses in terminally ill patients: prospective cohort study Commentary: Why do doctors overestimate? Commentary: Prognoses should be based on proved indices not intuition. *BMJ*. 2000;320(7233):469-473.

47. Organization NH. 1992 Stats show continued growth in programs and patients. *NHO Newsline*. 1993;3:1-2.

48. Lamont EB, Christakis NA. Prognostic disclosure to patients with cancer near the end of life. *Ann Intern Med*. 2001;134(12):1096-1105. PubMed PMID: 11412049.

49. Ryan CJ, Smith MR, Fizazi K, et al. Abiraterone acetate plus prednisone versus placebo plus prednisone in chemotherapy-naive men with metastatic castration-resistant prostate cancer (COU-AA-302): final overall survival analysis of a randomised, double-blind, placebo-controlled phase 3 study. *Lancet Oncol*. 2015;16(2):152-160.

50. Fizazi K, Scher HI, Molina A, et al. Abiraterone acetate for treatment of metastatic castration-resistant prostate cancer: final overall survival analysis of the COU-AA-301 randomised, double-blind, placebo-controlled phase 3 study. *Lancet Oncol*. 2012;13(10):983-992.

51. Cabot RC, Harris NL, Rosenberg ES, et al. Increased survival with enzalutamide in prostate cancer after chemotherapy. *N Eng J Med*. 2012;367(13):1187-1197.

52. Beer TM, Armstrong AJ, Rathkopf DE, et al. Enzalutamide in metastatic prostate cancer before chemotherapy. *N Engl J Med*. 2014;371(5):424-433.

53. Parker C, Nilsson S, Heinrich D, et al. Alpha emitter radium-223 and survival in metastatic prostate cancer. *N Engl J Med*. 2013;369(3):213-223.

54. Sahgal A, Aoyama H, Kocher M, et al. Phase 3 trials of stereotactic radiosurgery with or without whole-brain radiation therapy for 1 to 4 brain metastases: individual patient data meta-analysis. *Int J Radiat Oncol Biol Phys*. 2015;91(4):710-717.

55. Salpeter SR, Malter DS, Luo EJ, et al. Systematic review of cancer presentations with a median survival of six months or less. *J Palliat Med*. 2012;15(2):175-185.

56. Fukuoka M, Wu Y-L, Thongprasert S, et al. Biomarker analyses and final overall survival results from a phase III, randomized, open-label, first-line study of gefitinib versus carboplatin/paclitaxel in clinically selected patients with advanced non–small-cell lung cancer in Asia (IPASS). *J Clin Oncol*. 2011;29(21):2866-2874.

57. Gupta S, Tran T, Luo W, et al. Machine-learning prediction of cancer survival: a retrospective study using electronic administrative records and a cancer registry. *BMJ Open*. 2014;4(3):e004007.

58. Campos S, Presutti R, Zhang L, et al. Elderly patients with painful bone metastases should be offered palliative radiotherapy. *Int J Radiat Oncol Biol Phys*. 2010;76(5):1500-1506.

59. Westhoff PG, de Graeff A, Reyners AK, et al. Effect of age on response to palliative radiotherapy and quality of life in patients with painful bone metastases. *Radiother Oncol*. 2014;111(2):264-269.

60. Dennis K, Wong K, Zhang L, et al. Palliative radiotherapy for bone metastases in the last 3 months of life: worthwhile or futile? *Clin Oncol (R Coll Radiol)*. 2011;23(10):709-715.

61. Meeuse JJ, van der Linden YM, van Tienhoven G, et al. Efficacy of radiotherapy for painful bone metastases during the last 12 weeks of life: results from the Dutch Bone Metastasis Study. *Cancer*. June 1, 2010;116(11):2716-2725. PubMed PMID: 20225326.

62. Meeuse JJ, van der Linden YM, van Tienhoven G, et al. Efficacy of radiotherapy for painful bone metastases during the last 12 weeks of life. *Cancer*. 2010;116(11):2716-2725.

63. Rades D, Fehlauer F, Schulte R, et al. Prognostic factors for local control and survival after radiotherapy of metastatic spinal cord compression. *J Clin Oncol*. 2006;24(21):3388-3393.

64. Rades D, Lange M, Veninga T, et al. Final results of a prospective study comparing the local control of short-course and long-course radiotherapy for metastatic spinal cord compression. *Int J Radiat Oncol Biol Phys*. 2011;79(2):524-530.

65. Maranzano E, Trippa F, Casale M, et al. 8 Gy single-dose radiotherapy is effective in metastatic spinal cord compression: results of a phase III randomized multicentre Italian trial. *Radiother Oncol*. 2009;93(2):174-179.

66. Rades D, Panzner A, Rudat V, et al. Dose escalation of radiotherapy for metastatic spinal cord compression (MSCC) in patients with relatively favorable survival prognosis. *Strahlenther Onkol*. 2011;187(11):729-735.

67. Brown PD, Jaeckle K, Ballman KV, et al. Effect of radiosurgery alone vs radiosurgery with whole brain radiation therapy on cognitive function in patients with 1 to 3 brain metastases: a randomized clinical trial. *JAMA*. 2016;316(4):401-409.

68. Windsor A, Koh E-S, Allen S, et al. Poor outcomes after whole brain radiotherapy in patients with brain metastases: results from an international multicentre cohort study. *Clin Oncol (R Coll Radiol)*. 2013;25(11):674-680.

69. Mulvenna PM, Nankivell MG, Barton R, et al., editors. Whole brain radiotherapy for brain metastases from non-small lung cancer: quality of life (QoL) and overall survival (OS) results from the UK Medical Research Council QUARTZ randomised clinical trial (ISRCTN 3826061). ASCO Annual Meeting Proceedings; 2015; Chicago, IL.

3 Bone Metastases

Pei Shuen Lim and Peter J. Hoskin

INTRODUCTION

Approximately 50% of the workload in a radiation therapy (RT) department is comprised of palliative work, of which the most common indication is bone metastases.[1] Bone is the third most frequent site of metastatic disease following lung and liver.[2] The incidence of bone metastases is highest in breast and prostate cancer, where up to 80% of patients have evidence of metastatic bone disease at autopsy studies.[3] Other tumors that frequently metastasize to the bones include lung, kidney, and thyroid cancers, with an incidence of around 30%.[4]

Bone metastases affect the axial skeleton more commonly than the appendicular skeleton. It has been suggested that the reason for this is that the axial skeleton contains a higher proportion of red marrow, which has an increased blood supply, stem cells, and extracellular matrix, therefore promoting tumor growth. The distribution of bone metastases in the skeleton has been described in this descending order of frequency: lumbar spine, thoracic spine, pelvis, ribs, femur, skull, cervical spine, humerus.[2] In the long bones, proximal regions are involved earlier than distal regions.

Symptoms from bone metastases can cause significant morbidity, affecting the patient's overall quality of life and function. Local symptoms include pain, pathological fracture, spinal cord compression, and nerve root compression. Systemic complications can also occur such as hypercalcemia and bone marrow suppression secondary to marrow infiltration. The main goals of palliative treatment in this setting are pain relief and function preservation.

RADIATION THERAPY FOR BONE METASTASES

Local Bone Pain

External beam radiation therapy (EBRT) offers excellent local palliation for painful bone metastases leading to an improvement in quality of life with little toxicity.[5,6] The median time to onset of pain relief is around 3 weeks.[7] Overall pain relief is obtained in 60% to 80% of patients and 25% of patients achieve complete response after initial EBRT.[8] The median duration of response varies

TABLE 3.1 Mirels' Score for Assessing Risk of Pathological Fracture. A Total Score of Greater Than 8 Suggests the Need for Prophylactic Internal Fixation Prior to Radiation Therapy[12]

	Score		
Parameter	**1**	**2**	**3**
Site	Upper limb	Lower limb	Peri-trochanter
Pain	Mild	Moderate	Severe
Lesion	Blastic	Mixed	Lytic
Size (of shaft)	<1/3	1/3–2/3	>2/3

between 11 and 24 weeks.[9] The net pain response is an objective method of assessing duration of pain relief relative to the survival of a patient, which has been found to be between 63% and 71%.[10,11]

Pathological Fracture

Metastases weaken the stability of the bone, leading to an increased risk of pathological fracture especially in weight bearing bones. The morbidity and mortality of a fracture are significant. Therefore, accurate prediction of the risk of an impending pathological fracture is crucial—not only to prevent the morbidity of a fracture in high-risk patients but also to avoid overtreatment with unnecessary prophylactic osteosynthesis in a group of patients with limited life expectancies, who may benefit from simple RT or bisphosphonates if the lesions are at lower risk of fracturing.

The Mirels' score is based on four criteria: pain, size, site, and nature, to form a 12-point scale to predict the risk of impending fracture (Table 3.1).[12] This scoring system has been found to overestimate the risk in some studies.[13,14] The Dutch Bone Metastases study group recommends the use of a simple radiographic parameter measuring the largest axial cortical involvement (Lcort).[15] If the Lcort is less than 30 mm, RT is recommended. If the Lcort is more than 30 mm, prophylactic surgical osteosynthesis should be considered followed by RT if appropriate.

DOSE FRACTIONATION

Single fraction (SF) and multiple fraction (MF) RT schedules for the treatment of uncomplicated bone metastases have been shown to be equivalent. Four large meta-analyses, including an update in 2012, reviewing multiple

TABLE 3.2 Summary of the Outcomes and Adverse Events Shown in
Meta-Analyses of Randomized Clinical Trials Comparing Single Fraction (SF)
Versus Multiple Fraction (MF) Radiation Therapy Regimens

Meta-Analysis	No of Trials		Overall Response Rate (%)	Complete Response Rate (%)	Reirradiation Rate (%)	Pathological Fracture Rate (%)
Chow et al. (2012)[8] (update of Chow et al., 2007)[16]	25	SF	60	23	20	3.3
		MF	61	24	8	3.0
Sze et al. (2004)[17]	12	SF	60	34	21.5	3
		MF	59	32	7.4	1.6
Wu et al. (2003)[9]	8	SF	62.1	33.4	21	N/A
		MF	58.7	32.3	6.4	N/A

randomized controlled trials has consistently confirmed this result (Table 3.2).
Overall and complete response rates were similar. No additional benefit was
seen with higher total doses of RT regardless of tumor type, expected survival,
or site of metastases. Although retreatment rates with SF seem to be higher
at 20% compared to 8% after MF, these differences are subject to bias as the
option of retreatment was at the discretion of the treating clinician.

SF RT is convenient, efficient, and effective.[18] It reduces unnecessary hospital visits, particularly benefiting patients who are facing end of life, are limited by pain, or have poor performance status. It is also cost effective for a RT
department, allowing appropriate utilization of resources.[19,20]

The American Society for Radiation Oncology (ASTRO)[6] and American
College of Radiology (ACR)[21,22] have published treatment guidelines for bone
metastases recognizing the benefits of SF. 8 Gy has been found to be the
optimal SF dose in achieving response when randomized against 4 Gy SF.[23]
Recommended MF schedules by ASTRO are 30 Gy in 10 fractions, 24 Gy in
6 fractions, and 20 Gy in 5 fractions.

In 2012, the National Quality Forum (NQF), a U.S.-based organization
that reviews quality metrics, has endorsed a performance measure on the use
of EBRT for bone metastases based on the ASTRO guidelines, supporting shorter
RT schedules.[24] This measure is aimed at addressing the gap in dose fractionation treatment variations among clinicians[25] and preventing the overuse of
radiation therapy. The "Choosing Wisely" campaign is an initiative targeted at
reducing unnecessary tests and treatments in the U.S. health care system. They

have recommended the use of SF and discouraged the routine use of extended fractionation schedules (>10 fractions) for the palliation of bone metastases.[26,27]

Despite extensive evidence supporting the use of SF and published guidance, international surveys still show that SF is still underutilized globally.[25,28] One reason against the use of SF is the higher retreatment rates associated with it.[29] The trial protocols left the option to retreat up to clinician discretion. They were not blinded to initial dose fractionation schedules, leading to biased results. Clinicians were more likely to offer retreatment after SF RT as they would still be within radiation tolerance after SF and there is the possibility that clinicians may have felt that SF treatment was insufficient.[30]

Some argue for the use of MF in order to achieve longer term responses in patients with better prognoses. A subgroup analysis of patients with more favorable prognoses, surviving more than 1 year, in the Dutch Bone Metastases study demonstrated no additional benefit in the duration of response after initial response with MF compared to SF, which was around 29 to 30 weeks in both arms.[31] Oncologists in general tend to be more optimistic in predicting survival.[32,33] It is important to remember that symptomatic pain relief is the main goal of treatment for the majority of patients with metastatic bone disease, not tumor control. For patients with true oligometastatic disease and good performance status, MF or stereotactic RT may be a reasonable option.

For neuropathic pain, only a single trial so far has addressed fractionation.[34] The authors concluded that SF was neither as effective, nor worse than MF. The duration of response was slightly better after MF. Further trials in this area should therefore be carried out to validate these results.[35]

Higher total doses, 20 to 30 Gy, are considered appropriate for complicated bony lesions with extensive soft-tissue components or lesions with impending fractures, which are surgically inoperable.[36] Increased tumor control with higher doses allows the induction of bone mineralization. However, this process may take up to several months to occur. It is therefore imperative to carefully select patients who are offered MF to ensure that the clinical benefits are not offset by the side effects and prolonged inconvenience of fractionated treatment.

REIRRADIATION

Improvements in systemic and supportive therapies have increased the life expectancies of patients with bone metastases. More patients are therefore outliving the duration of benefits from their initial RT. Approximately 50% of patients who responded to initial treatment experience pain relapse within 1 year from treatment.[7]

Two systematic reviews have confirmed the efficacy of reirradiation of painful bone metastases.[37,38] Repeat radiation is indicated for patients in these three scenarios:

1. No pain relief after initial radiation
2. Partial response after initial radiation who may receive benefit from further doses
3. Pain relapse after satisfactory response to initial radiation

It is recommended that a 4-week period should be given before considering reirradiation to allow enough time to observe the response from the initial treatment.[8]

The NCIG CTG SC20 is a prospective randomized trial that investigated dose fractionation schedules of reirradiation. 8 Gy SF was found to be non-inferior and less toxic compared to 20 Gy MF.[39] The overall response rate for reirradiation was 48% regardless of response to initial therapy, with 11% to 14% achieving complete response in the per-protocol analysis. Sixty-eight percent of patients reported an improvement in their quality of life.

A pooled analysis looking at overall response rates in patients who underwent both initial treatment and retreatment demonstrated that there was no difference in outcome between different fractionation schedules: SF/SF, SF/MF, MF/SF, and MF/MF. All schedules had overall response rates within 2% of each other.[40]

When retreating spinal metastases, spinal cord tolerance must be considered. Cord tolerance is still a subject of uncertainty. The risk of myelopathy is low if the interval between treatments is no less than 6 months and the total cumulative biological effective dose (BED) is kept below 135.5 Gy_2 ($\alpha/\beta = 2$).[41] QUANTEC recommends using cord α/β at 0.87 and estimates a 0.2% risk of myelopathy at 50 Gy EQD2. Cord recovery is at least 25% at 6 months after initial treatment.[42] A dose of 30 Gy in 10 fractions delivers 40.6 Gy EQD2, 20 Gy in 5 fractions delivers 34 Gy EQD2, and an 8 Gy SF delivers 24.8 Gy EQD2. (EQD2 formula = $(n{\cdot}d\ [1 + d/\alpha/\beta])/1 + 2/\alpha/\beta$; n = number of fractions, d = dose per fraction.) This illustrates how a higher dose given at initial treatment may preclude the patient from being offered retreatment at a later date, as it may exceed cord tolerance.

CHOICE OF TREATMENT AND PROGNOSIS

Patients with painful bone metastases have a median survival of 7 to 9 months.[31]

Even in the group of patients who were reirradiated in the SC20 trial, median overall survival was between 9.3 and 9.7 months, which is likely to be an overestimate of the unselected population.[39] Survival is dependent on type of primary tumor, with breast and prostate cancer extending over years, while lung cancer is measured in months.[4,43] The presence of visceral metastases is associated with a worse prognosis.

With no strong evidence advocating one schedule over another, the choice of treatment needs to be made together with the patient and her family, taking into account symptoms, life expectancy, quality of life, cost, and expectations. An initial SF treatment followed by a repeat SF if necessary is a more pragmatic and cost-effective approach than upfront MF RT. The cost of two SF treatments is lower than MF, even after taking into account the additional costs of medications and hospital admissions.[20,44]

TREATMENT PLANNING

General Radiation Therapy Planning and Delivery

The following is a stepwise approach in the work up of delivering RT to bone metastases:

- Gather and interpret all relevant clinical information
  - History, examination, and assessment—Where is the pain if there are multiple sites of bony metastases on imaging? What stage of the disease is the patient at? Are there any systemic treatment options available? What is his performance status?
  - Diagnostic imaging—MRI, CT, bone scan, plain radiographs
- Consent
- Simulation
  - Fluoroscopy or CT planning
    - A conventional fluoroscopy simulator is being replaced with CT simulation in most departments as CT images allow optimal anatomical visualization of target volumes and critical structures. Virtual simulation is adequate for straightforward cases. Formal planning with dose distribution assessment may be beneficial for tumors that are in close proximity to organs at risk, such as large para-spinal masses, where there may be an increased risk of toxicity with large doses per fraction.
  - Patient positioning
    - The patient should be placed in a comfortable, reproducible position that can be maintained for at least 10 to 15 minutes. The need for adequate analgesia must be anticipated and given.
    - Most sites can be treated supine, with exceptions being the ribs, clavicle, and skull when treated with direct electrons; it may be necessary to be positioned semisupine, lateral, or prone.

- ▪ Arm positioning
  - • Thorax—above head or by sides depending on the angle of beam entry
  - • Pelvis—arms by sides or across chest if using more than two fields
  - • Humerus—arms abducted, elbows flexed, hands on hips
- • Immobilization to aid reproducibility
  - ▪ Leg or ankle stocks, headrest, foam wedges
  - ▪ Shoulder retractors can be used to bring shoulders down and away from the lateral fields used to treat the cervical spine region
  - ▪ Thermoplastic shells can be used for head and neck immobilization
  - ▪ Immobilization tools used should be kept as simple and practical as possible to allow seamless reproducibility, as most of these patients are in pain and would not tolerate elaborate set-up sessions
- ▪ Target volume definition
  - • Treatment volumes should be based on symptoms, not just radiological findings.
  - • Field edges represent the 50% isodose line.
  - • Symptomatic lesions should be adequately included within the 90% isodose region, taking into consideration internal organ movement and set-up variation. A 1- to 2-cm margin is generally sufficient for this purpose.
  - • Field edges should ideally coincide with anatomical borders to allow for subsequent matching of adjacent fields if future treatments are required. Borders commonly used are the intervertebral spaces, vertebral body, transverse processes, pubic symphysis, lesser trochanter, and acetabulum.
  - • Structures such as joint spaces and vertebral body should be fully covered.
  - • Balance between disease treated and toxicity should always be considered.
- ▪ Dose prescription
  - • Single applied fields prescribed to a particular depth or parallel opposed fields prescribed to the midplane dose (MPD) using 6-10-MV photons.
  - • For 3D conformal plans, dose is prescribed to 100% at the International Commission on Radiation Units and Measurements (ICRU) reference point.
  - • For superficial lesions (ribs, scapula, skull), direct electrons or orthovoltage beams can be used.
- ▪ Verification and image guidance
  - • This step is important especially with hypofractionated schedules. KV portal imaging or cone beam CT can be used to verify patient set up and guide positional corrections prior to treatment delivery.

RADIATION THERAPY PLANNING TO THE SPINE

The whole vertebra containing the lesion should be treated. One vertebra superior and inferior to the involved site should be included, with field edges at the intervertebral space. This ensures the vertebra intended for treatment is adequately covered within the 90% isodose level as the field borders represent the 50% isodose. Lateral borders are the transverse processes and should encompass any paravertebral disease extension.

Several cases and figures are presented to illustrate radiation planning for bone metastases.

Case 3.1: Upper Cervical Spine Radiation Therapy

A 60-year-old, previously fit lady presented with a painful C2 spinal lesion from metastatic lung cancer (Figure 3.1a). Her Karnofsky performance score (KPS) was 60 due to the severity of neuropathic pain. Parallel-opposed lateral beams prescribed to the MPD were used for the upper cervical spine to minimize toxicity to the oral cavity and pharynx (Figure 3.1b). Choice of dose fractionation was 20 Gy in 5 fractions, as there was a neuropathic component to her pain and due to the close proximity of the RT fields to surrounding critical structures (brain stem, cerebellum, parotids).

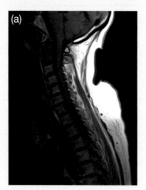 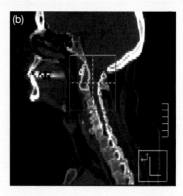

FIGURE 3.1 (a) MRI T1 weighted sagittal view demonstrating complete infiltration of the C2 vertebra. (b) Lateral treatment field. Blue lines: treatment field edges, Green line: contour of C2 lesion.

Case 3.2: Lower Cervical Spine–Thoracic Spine Radiation Therapy

This patient underwent spinal decompression and C6–T4 fixation for soft-tissue bone metastases at T1-2 secondary to early chemotherapy naïve metastatic prostate carcinoma. Parallel-opposed anterior and posterior fields are used in this situation, as the shoulders will be in the way of lateral beams (Figure 3.2). Acceptable dose fractionation: 20 Gy in 5 fractions, 30 Gy in 10 fractions.[6] There is little data on the use of SF in the postoperative setting but can be considered in patients with limited life expectancies and poor mobility.

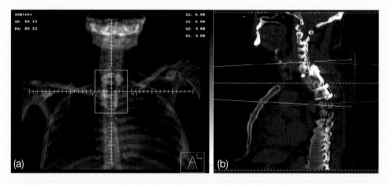

FIGURE 3.2 (a) Treatment field on the digital reconstructed radiograph (DRR) of the planning scan. (b) Sagittal view of planning CT with anterior and posterior beams encompassing metal work.

Case 3.3: Thoracic Spine in a Patient With Diffuse Metastases

A 70-year-old lady with end-stage metastatic breast cancer complains of midthoracic pain, requiring high-dose opiates. Her bone scan (Figure 3.3a) shows diffuse spinal metastases. In this case, it is useful to perform a clinical examination to identify and mark areas of pain prior to the planning CT scan (Figure 3.3b). Marking was done with radio-opaque ball bearings so that it was visible on the CT scan. 8 Gy SF was used.

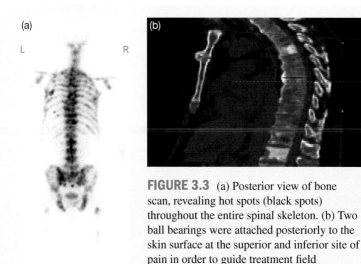

(a)

L   R

(b)

FIGURE 3.3 (a) Posterior view of bone scan, revealing hot spots (black spots) throughout the entire spinal skeleton. (b) Two ball bearings were attached posteriorly to the skin surface at the superior and inferior site of pain in order to guide treatment field application.

Case 3.4: Treatment of the Lumbar and Sacral Spine

For the lower spine, a single applied posterior photon field prescribed to the depth of the anterior spinal canal is commonly used. A 65-year-old man with metastatic prostate cancer presented with lower back pain. His bone scan (not shown) demonstrated sclerotic lesions from thoracic vertebra T12 through lumbar vertebra L3. Figure 3.4a shows a posterior–anterior (PA) field treating the lower thoracic and lumbar spine only. In contrast, if this patient had pain corresponding to lesions in the lumbar and sacral spine, the width of treatment field is extended to cover the sacrum (Figure 3.4b). Shielding is used to minimize bowel toxicity in the lumbar area. Lateral borders include the sacro-iliac joints with the inferior border at the top of the acetabulum. Figure 3.4c demonstrates isodose curves from a patient treated with 8 Gy in a SF from L3 through the sacrum for painful bone metastasis using an anterior–posterior (AP)–PA beam arrangement.

Given the presence of other adjacent bone disease, a half-beam block was used superiorly. This can aid in the matching of adjacent fields if adjacent vertebral lesions become painful.

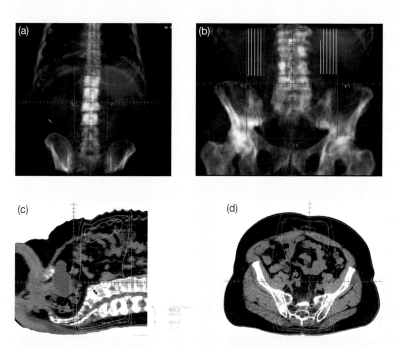

FIGURE 3.4 (a) T11–L4 treatment field on DRR. (b) Lumbar-sacral spade treatment field on DRR with multileaf collimator (MLC) shielding. (c) and (d): Isodose curves in the sagittal and axial planes for a patient treated from L3 through the sacrum with a half-beam block superiorly.

RADIATION THERAPY FOR NONSPINE METASTASES

Several cases and figures illustrate radiation treatment planning for treatment of nonspine bone metastasis.

Case 3.5: Radiation Treatment of the Hemipelvis

An 80-year-old lady was admitted with worsening hip pain limiting her mobility. Further investigation revealed a soft-tissue mass in the left iliac bone secondary to a primary lung carcinoma. She was transferred for same day RT planning and treatment with 8 Gy SF to the hemipelvis (Figure 3.5). In this scenario, given her poor performance status and poor prognosis with primary lung malignancy, the chances of offering any systemic treatment are slim. SF would be highly appropriate to alleviate her symptoms in the first instance, although it is a large soft-tissue lesion. The RT field was extended to cover the lumbar spine, as there were other lesions, but shielded inferior-medially up to the pubic symphysis to minimize dose to the bowels as shown in Figure 3.5c and d. AP parallel-opposed beams were used.

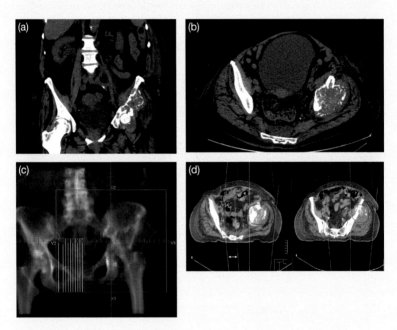

FIGURE 3.5 (a) and (b) Coronal and axial view of diagnostic CT imaging with large destructive lesion in the left iliac bone. (c) Hemipelvis treatment field on DRR. (d) Axial view of planning CT scan demonstrating bowels with and without shielding (double arrow in yellow: shielded area, red contour: destructive lesion).

Case 3.6: Radiation Treatment of the Femur

A 59-year-old man with end-stage chemotherapy refractory prostate cancer has a painful lesion seen on the bone scan in the lesser trochanter of the femur (Figure 3.6a). Figure 3.6b illustrates the treatment fields. The Mirels' score assessing risk of pathological fracture for this patient was 6 (refer to Table 3.1); hence, no surgical intervention was required. This patient was at the end stage of his disease, therefore an 8 Gy SF was given. Despite a slightly lower trend of pathological fractures seen with MF RT in the meta-analyses data discussed earlier (refer to Table 3.2), the differences were not statistically significant and were not primary end points of many of the trials reviewed.

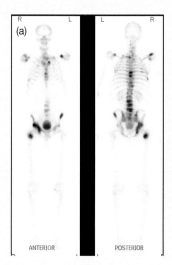
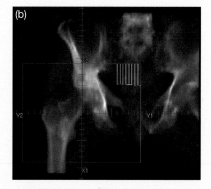

FIGURE 3.6 (a) Bone scan demonstrating lesion seen in lesser trochanter and acetabulum.
(b) Treatment field shown on DRR.

Case 3.7: Postoperative Radiation Treatment of the Femur

A 60-year-old man with newly diagnosed prostate cancer presented with pain in his right knee. An MRI of his femurs revealed a 3-cm-long metastases involving more than 50% the width of his right midfemoral shaft (Figure 3.7a). Given that hormone naïve prostate cancer patients carry a survival of a few years, prophylactic surgical internal fixation was performed as this lesion was at high risk of pathological fracture. He had postoperative RT with a 20 Gy in 5 fractions schedule (Figure 3.7b). The ACR guidelines recommend MF in this setting with the intent of eradicating as much disease as possible.[45] 30 Gy in 10 fractions is also acceptable. As mentioned earlier, there is little data published on the use of SF postoperatively.

There are two schools of thought as to what needs to be covered in the treatment volume, with not much evidence to support one over the other:

1. The entire bone as the marrow may be contaminated postoperatively.
2. The entire prosthesis only as it is the area most at risk of tumor regrowth.

As the field is long and encompasses the entire femur, it is ideal to preserve a "corridor" of normal tissue medially for lymphatic drainage. The joint spaces are avoided.

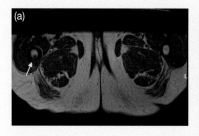 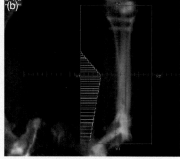

FIGURE 3.7 (a) Diagnostic MRI of the femurs. Tumor (yellow arrow) is invading the posterior cortex of the right femur and involves 50% of the width of the shaft. (b) Postoperative treatment field encompasses the length of the femur. Shielding of the "soft-tissue corridor" is done to reduce the risk of lymphedema. Note that the patient was scanned toe first toward the CT machine in order to scan the full length of his femur (normally head first).

Case 3.8: Radiation Treatment of the Humerus

A 59-year-old man with newly diagnosed lung cancer presented with pain in his right shoulder. Bone scan is shown in Figure 3.8a. Figure 3.8b shows treatment field for a lesion in the right proximal humerus. The shoulder joint is fully encompassed in the field. This patient was treated with 8 Gy in a single fraction. He experienced a pain flare that began within minutes of radiation therapy and was relieved with ibuprofen. The pain for which he was treated began to dissipate during the pain flare.

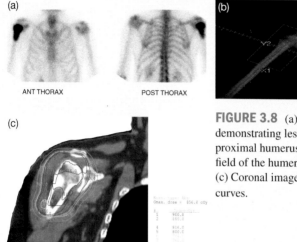

ANT THORAX   POST THORAX

FIGURE 3.8 (a) Bone scan demonstrating lesion in right proximal humerus. (b) Treatment field of the humerus on DRR. (c) Coronal image with isodose curves.

Case 3.9: Radiation Treatment of the Ribs

A 53-year-old woman with breast cancer presented with a superficial soft-tissue mass eroding into the ribs and sternum (Figure 3.9). The depth is 4 cm; a direct 12-MeV electron beam applied perpendicular to the skin surface will sufficiently treat the lesion. A more generous margin is usually given when using electrons to account for scatter, but should be balanced with the increased area subjected to skin toxicity. A direct photon field would cause unnecessary lung toxicity. A dose of 8 Gy SF would be appropriate. For more lateral rib lesions, tangential photon beams can be used.

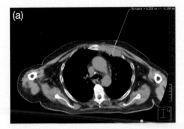 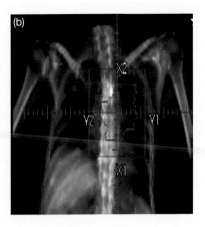

FIGURE 3.9 (a) Axial view of planning CT scan showing depth of lesion from skin surface. (b) Contour of lesion and treatment field of electron on DRR.

Wide field hemibody RT can offer good palliation for widespread bone metastases.[46] However, in the era of improved systemic therapies such as bisphosphonates and radioisotopes, the need for this technique is becoming increasingly rare.

TOXICITY AND SYMPTOM MANAGEMENT

The toxicity of RT is dependent on the irradiated body site, treatment volume, and total dose given. Acute side effects can occur during the treatment course and can last for a few weeks after completion. Common effects are fatigue, local skin reaction, nausea, diarrhea, or mucositis, if mucosal surfaces are in the irradiated fields. Three trials reviewed in the most recent meta-analysis of MF versus SF reported greater acute toxicities in patients who received MF.[29] Antiemetics for nausea and analgesia for pain can be useful. Around 30% to 40% of patients experience the "pain flare" phenomenon, where a transient increase in pain is observed over the irradiated site 1 to 5 days after completing treatment. The prophylactic use of dexamethasone 8 mg daily taken 1 hour prior to RT for 5 days has been found to be effective in a placebo controlled randomized controlled trial.[47] In the same study, dexamethasone was also found to reduce nausea. If a pain flare occurs, adequate analgesia must be offered. Short-term dexamethasone use should be considered, but with caution in patients with preexisting diabetes.

Late side effects occur months to years after RT and are dependent more on the dose per fraction and total dose delivered. The main concern is the risk of myelopathy if the spinal cord is encompassed in the treatment field.

As long as the dose tolerances of the "organs at risk" are respected, RT is safe. Patients with bone metastases generally do not live long enough to develop late toxicities. Modern highly conformal RT technologies such as intensity modulated RT and stereotactic body RT may have an emerging role in minimizing dose to adjacent normal structures. Stereotactic body RT allows treatment to be delivered with high accuracy to spinal metastases whilst avoiding dose to the spinal cord. This is increasingly used in patients with low volume oligometastatic disease with good prognosis histological tumor types when tumor ablation may be the aim of treatment.

SUMMARY

RT is a well-recognized modality for palliative treatment of bone metastases. 8 Gy SF as an initial treatment or retreatment is highly efficacious, cost-effective, and convenient. Choice of dose fractionation needs to be based on the holistic assessment of tumor characteristics, patient fitness, patient choice, and social circumstances, to avoid unnecessary and time-consuming interventions and toxicity for a patient with an incurable, advanced malignancy and with a limited life expectancy.

CLINICAL PEARLS

- Palliation is the goal rather than tumor control in most cases.
- Indications for RT: local pain, impending pathological fracture, postorthopedic surgical intervention.
- SF and MF for initial RT are equally efficacious. Retreatment rates are higher in SF, but results are biased.
- SF is also noninferior to MF in the reirradiation setting and less toxic.
- 8 Gy is the optimal dose for SF RT.

SELF-ASSESSMENT

Case 3.5: Self-Assessment Questions 1 to 4

A 50-year-old man with metastatic squamous cell carcinoma of the tonsil has recently progressed on systemic chemotherapy. He received radical chemoradiotherapy to the tonsil and bilateral neck 2 years ago. He complains of worsening right shoulder and back pain. A diagnostic CT scan revealed soft-tissue metastases destroying his right scapula and T3 vertebra. He had missed two RT planning appointments due to pain.

1. Outline the lesions seen on the CT planning scan (Figure 3.10a and b).

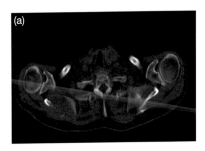 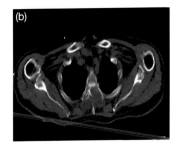

FIGURE 3.10 (a) and (b): Axial planning CT images. (c) DRR with contours of soft-tissue lesion. (d) and (e) Axial CT planning images with soft tissue abnormalities outlined. (f) Treatment field on DRR for Assessment 1.

2. What dose fractionation would you offer and why? What other factors would you take into consideration?

3. Draw the treatment field(s) on the DRR shown in Figure 3.10c.

4. What supportive medications would you offer?

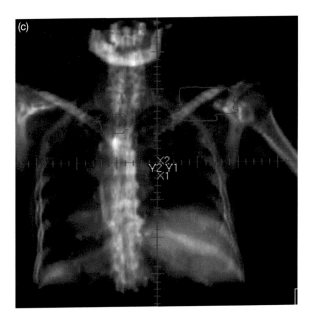

Answers

1. Figure 3.10d and 3.10e, showing contours of soft-tissue lesion in right scapula and vertebrae.

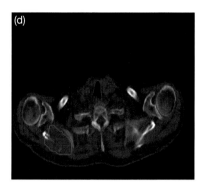
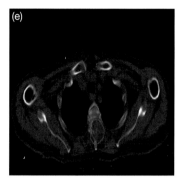

2. It is good practice to review doses and treatment fields of any previous RT received. This man received radical doses of RT to his neck. Upon review of his previous treatment fields, his spinal cord was treated up to the level of T1 and received a maximum cumulative dose of 45 Gy in 30 fractions, which equates to a BED of 78 Gy_2. (BED formula = $n \cdot d \, [1 + d/\alpha/\beta]$; n = number of fractions, d = dose per fraction.) The BED will be slightly higher with chemoradiotherapy. Accounting for his previous treatment and possible overlap of fields, his cumulative BED with 8 Gy SF would be 78 Gy_2 + 40 Gy_2 = 118 Gy_2. Allowing for some spinal cord recovery over 2 years (25%–50% recovery), the spinal cord would be in tolerance.

   Given the patient's poor prognosis with chemotherapy-resistant metastatic head and neck malignancy, coupled with severe pain limiting his mobility, 8 Gy SF would be highly appropriate. Same day planning and treatment delivery would be more convenient for the patient, saving the patient an unnecessary hospital visit.

3. Both lesions were treated using one field (Figure 3.10f) as they were in close proximity to each other. If two separate fields were to be used, there would be the possibility of overlap due to beam divergence. Note that the whole shoulder joint is included. A single direct posterior beam using 6-MV photons was used, prescribed to a 5-cm depth. Shielding was used as a conservative measure superiorly to avoid unnecessary toxicity to the previously treated spine.

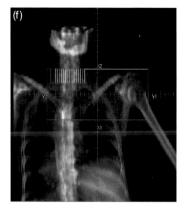

4. Dexamethasone, analgesia, and antiemetics.

Case 3.6: Self-Assessment Questions 5 and 6

A 65-year-old man currently on antiandrogen therapy for metastatic prostate cancer presented with headaches and right facial pain. A diagnostic CT scan revealed a bone metastases in the right sphenoid bone (Figure 3.11a).

5. Draw your treatment fields on DRR in Figure 3.11b.

6. What dose fractionation would you offer and why?

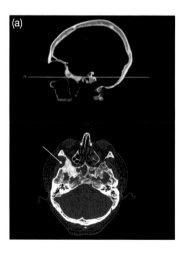

FIGURE 3.11 (a) Yellow arrow pointing toward right sphenoid bone metastases. (b) DRR for Assessment 2. (c) Axial, sagittal, and coronal views of lateral beams on planning CT scan.

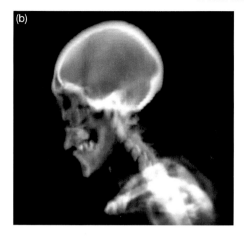

Answers

5. Two lateral opposed fields (Figure 3.11c) with a collimator twist angle at 105° is used to treat this man's base of skull. The beam's edges are positioned well away from the lens anteriorly.

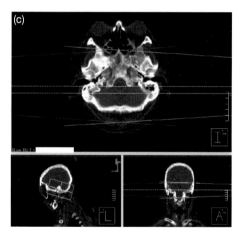

6. 20 Gy in 5 fractions was offered to the patient as the treatment fields involve the brainstem and cerebellum.

REFERENCES

1. Chow E, Danjoux C, Wong R, et al. Palliation of bone metastases: a survey of patterns of practice among Canadian radiation oncologists. *Radiother Oncol.* 2000;56(3):305-314.

2. Tubiana-Hulin M. Incidence, prevalence and distribution of bone metastases. Bone. 1991;12(suppl 1):S9-S10.
3. Galasko CS. Skeletal metastases. *Clin Orthop Relat Res*. 1986;210:18-30.
4. Coleman RE. Clinical features of metastatic bone disease and risk of skeletal morbidity. *Clin Cancer Res*. 2006;12(20 pt 2):6243s-6249s.
5. Zeng L, Chow E, Bedard G, et al. Quality of life after palliative radiation therapy for patients with painful bone metastases: results of an international study validating the EORTC QLQ-BM22. *Int J Radiat Oncol Biol Phys*. 2012;84(3):e337-e342.
6. Lutz S, Berk L, Chang E, et al. Palliative radiotherapy for bone metastases: an ASTRO evidence-based guideline. *Int J Radiat Oncol Biol Phys*. 2011;79(4):965-976.
7. Steenland E, Leer JW, van Houwelingen H, et al. The effect of a single fraction compared to multiple fractions on painful bone metastases: a global analysis of the Dutch Bone Metastasis Study. *Radiother Oncol*. 1999;52(2):101-109.
8. Chow E, Hoskin P, Mitera G, et al. Update of the international consensus on palliative radiotherapy endpoints for future clinical trials in bone metastases. *Int J Radiat Oncol Biol Phys*. 2012;82(5):1730-1737.
9. Wu JS, Wong R, Johnston M, et al. Meta-analysis of dose-fractionation radiotherapy trials for the palliation of painful bone metastases. *Int J Radiat Oncol Biol Phys*. 2003;55(3):594-605.
10. Foro Arnalot P, Fontanals AV, Galcerán JC, et al. Randomized clinical trial with two palliative radiotherapy regimens in painful bone metastases: 30 Gy in 10 fractions compared with 8 Gy in single fraction. *Radiother Oncol*. 2008;89(2):150-155.
11. Meeuse JJ, van der Linden YM, van Tienhoven G, et al. Efficacy of radiotherapy for painful bone metastases during the last 12 weeks of life: results from the Dutch Bone Metastasis Study. *Cancer*. 2010;116(11):2716-2725.
12. Mirels H. Metastatic disease in long bones. A proposed scoring system for diagnosing impending pathologic fractures. *Clin Orthop Relat Res*. 1989;(249):256-264.
13. Mac Niocaill RF, Quinlan JF, Stapleton RD, et al. Inter- and intra-observer variability associated with the use of the Mirels' scoring system for metastatic bone lesions. *Int Orthop*. 2011;35(1):83-86.
14. Damron TA, Ward WG. Risk of pathologic fracture: assessment. *Clin Orthop Relat Res*. 2003;(415 suppl):S208-S211.
15. van der Linden YM, Kroon HM, Dijkstra SP, et al. Simple radiographic parameter predicts fracturing in metastatic femoral bone lesions: results from a randomised trial. *Radiother Oncol*. 2003;69(1):21-31.
16. Chow E, Harris K, Fan G, et al. Palliative radiotherapy trials for bone metastases: a systematic review. *J Clin Oncol*. 2007;25(11):1423-1436.
17. Sze WM, Shelley M, Held I, Mason M. Palliation of metastatic bone pain: single fraction versus multifraction radiotherapy—a systematic review of the randomised trials. *Cochrane Database Syst Rev*. 2004;(2):CD004721.
18. Lutz ST, Chow EL, Hartsell WF, Konski AA. A review of hypofractionated palliative radiotherapy. *Cancer*. 2007;109(8):1462-1470.

19. Konski A, James J, Hartsell W, et al. Economic analysis of radiation therapy oncology group 97–14: multiple versus single fraction radiation treatment of patients with bone metastases. *Am J Clin Oncol*. 2009;32(4):423-428.

20. van den Hout WB, van der Linden YM, Steenland E, et al. Single- versus multiple-fraction radiotherapy in patients with painful bone metastases: cost-utility analysis based on a randomized trial. *J Natl Cancer Inst*. 2003;95(3):222-229.

21. Kim EY, Chapman TR, Ryu S, et al. ACR Appropriateness Criteria(R) non-spine bone metastases. *J Palliat Med*. 2015;18(1):11-17.

22. Expert Panel on Radiation Oncology-Bone M, Lo SS, Lutz ST, et al. ACR Appropriateness Criteria (R) spinal bone metastases. *J Palliat Med*. 2013;16(1):9-19.

23. Hoskin P, Rojas A, Fidarova E, et al. IAEA randomised trial of optimal single dose radiotherapy in the treatment of painful bone metastases. *Radiother Oncol*. 2015;116(1):10-14.

24. Forum NQ. *External Beam Radiotherapy for Bone Metastases (NQF #1822)*. 2012 [cited 2016 March 29]. Available from http://www.qualityforum.org/QPS/1822.

25. Fairchild A, Barnes E, Ghosh S, et al. International patterns of practice in palliative radiotherapy for painful bone metastases: evidence-based practice? *Int J Radiat Oncol Biol Phys*. 2009;75(5):1501-1510.

26. Fischberg D, Bull J, Casarett D, et al. Five things physicians and patients should question in hospice and palliative medicine. *J Pain Symptom Manage*. 2013;45(3):595-605.

27. Hahn C, Kavanagh B, Bhatnagar A, et al. Choosing wisely: the American Society for Radiation Oncology's top 5 list. *Pract Radiat Oncol*. 2014;4(6):349-355.

28. Chow E, Hahn CA, Lutz ST. Global reluctance to practice evidence-based medicine continues in the treatment of uncomplicated painful bone metastases despite level 1 evidence and practice guidelines. *Int J Radiat Oncol Biol Phys*. 2012;83(1):1-2.

29. Chow E, Zeng L, Salvo N, et al. Update on the systematic review of palliative radiotherapy trials for bone metastases. *Clin Oncol (R Coll Radiol)*. 2012;24(2):112-124.

30. van der Linden YM, Lok JJ, Steenland E. Single fraction radiotherapy is efficacious: a further analysis of the Dutch Bone Metastasis Study controlling for the influence of retreatment. *Int J Radiat Oncol Biol Phys*. 2004;59(2):528-537.

31. van der Linden YM, Steenland E, van Houwelingen HC. Patients with a favourable prognosis are equally palliated with single and multiple fraction radiotherapy: results on survival in the Dutch Bone Metastasis Study. *Radiother Oncol*. 2006;78(3):245-253.

32. Chow E, Davis L, Panzarella T. Accuracy of survival prediction by palliative radiation oncologists. *Int J Radiat Oncol Biol Phys*. 2005;61(3):870-873.

33. Hartsell WF, Desilvio M, Bruner DW. Can physicians accurately predict survival time in patients with metastatic cancer? Analysis of RTOG 97-14. *J Palliat Med*. 2008;11(5):723-728.

34. Roos DE, Turner SL, O'Brien PC, et al. Randomized trial of 8 Gy in 1 versus 20 Gy in 5 fractions of radiotherapy for neuropathic pain due to bone metastases (Trans-Tasman Radiation Oncology Group, TROG 96.05). *Radiother Oncol.* 2005;75(1):54-63.

35. Dennis K, Chow E, Roos D, et al. Should bone metastases causing neuropathic pain be treated with single-dose radiotherapy? *Clin Oncol (R Coll Radiol).* 2011;23(7):482-484.

36. Van der Linden YM, Dijkstra PD, Kroon HM, et al. Comparative analysis of risk factors for pathological fracture with femoral metastases. *J Bone Joint Surg Br.* 2004;86(4):566-573.

37. Wong E, Hoskin P, Bedard G, et al. Re-irradiation for painful bone metastases—a systematic review. *Radiother Oncol.* 2014;110(1):61-70.

38. Huisman M, van den Bosch MA, Wijlemans JW, et al. Effectiveness of reirradiation for painful bone metastases: a systematic review and meta-analysis. *Int J Radiat Oncol Biol Phys.* 2012;84(1):8-14.

39. Chow E, Van der Linden YM, Roos D, et al. Single versus multiple fractions of repeat radiation for painful bone metastases: a randomised, controlled, non-inferiority trial. *Lancet Oncol.* 2014;15(2):164-171.

40. Bedard G, Hoskin P, Chow E. Overall response rates to radiation therapy for patients with painful uncomplicated bone metastases undergoing initial treatment and retreatment. *Radiother Oncol.* 2014;112(1):125-127.

41. Nieder C, Grosu AL, Andratschke NH, Molls M. Proposal of human spinal cord reirradiation dose based on collection of data from 40 patients. *Int J Radiat Oncol Biol Phys.* 2005;61(3):851-855.

42. Kirkpatrick JP, van der Kogel AJ, Schultheiss TE. Radiation dose-volume effects in the spinal cord. *Int J Radiat Oncol Biol Phys.* 2010;76(3 suppl):S42-S49.

43. Yong M, Jensen AÖ, Jacobsen JB, et al. Survival in breast cancer patients with bone metastases and skeletal-related events: a population-based cohort study in Denmark (1999–2007). *Breast Cancer Res Treat.* 2011;129(2):495-503.

44. Pollicino CA, Turner SL, Roos DE, O'Brien PC. Costing the components of pain management: analysis of Trans-Tasman Radiation Oncology Group trial (TROG 96.05): one versus five fractions for neuropathic bone pain. *Radiother Oncol.* 2005;76(3):264-269.

45. Expert Panel on Radiation Oncology-Bone Metastases, Lutz ST, Lo, SS, et al. ACR Appropriateness Criteria(R) non-spine bone metastases. *J Palliat Med.* 2012;15(5):521-526.

46. Salazar OM, Rubin P, Hendrickson FR, et al. Single-dose half-body irradiation for palliation of multiple bone metastases from solid tumors. Final Radiation Therapy Oncology Group report. *Cancer.* 1986;58(1):29-36.

47. Chow E, Meyer RM, Ding K, et al. Dexamethasone in the prophylaxis of radiation-induced pain flare after palliative radiotherapy for bone metastases: a double-blind, randomised placebo-controlled, phase 3 trial. *Lancet Oncol.* 2015;16(15):1463-1472.

4

Malignant Spinal Cord Compression

Randy Li-Hung Wei and Kavita V. Dharmarajan

INTRODUCTION

Epidemiology

Malignant spinal cord compression (MSCC) occurs when a soft-tissue tumor or pathological fracture of the spinal column impinges on the spinal cord or its vascular supply. Diagnosis of MSCC occurs in 2.5% to 10% of cancer patients and requires prompt diagnosis and intervention to maximize the chances for preserving neurologic function.[1] More than 95% of MSCC are extramedullary and most common secondary to the anterior portion of the vertebral column. Tumor-related back pain is the most common presenting symptom with 83% to 95% of patients with this symptom at presentation.[2] This type of pain is usually worse at night or early morning, and improves with activity during the day. The pain improves with a trial of low-dose steroids (i.e., dexamethasone 12-mg daily).[3] Other common symptoms are lower extremity weakness, sensory deficits, and loss of autonomic function (bladder and bowel control).

Diagnosis and Management

In patients with a history of cancer, any sensory or motor changes should be immediately concerning for MSCC, since an earlier diagnosis results in improved treatment outcomes. First, a detailed history and focused physical neurological examination is required to document the progression, duration, and extent of sensory or motor loss.

Secondly, an MRI of the spine with contrast of affected area is the most sensitive and specific modality for the diagnosis of MSCC. Given concerns for skip lesions in 10% of patients, an MRI should be performed for the entire spine.[4] If the patient has not had any recent imaging or has a newly diagnosed MSCC, then a patient should undergo a CT of the chest, abdomen, and pelvis because the majority of patients with MSCC have visceral and skeletal metastasis. Thirdly, an urgent surgical evaluation of the patient should be obtained, to assess spinal instability and possible surgical debulking and stabilization. The spinal instability neoplastic score (SINS) is a standardized and validated classification system to assess tumor-related instability that includes six individual component scores: spine location, pain, lesion bone quality, radiographic spinal alignment, vertebral body collapse, and posterolateral involvement of spinal elements.[5] A SINS score of 0 to 6 denotes stability, 7 to 12 denotes possibly impending, and 13 to 18 denotes instability. Surgical consult is warranted for patients with scores of 7 or greater (Table 4.1).

Treatment requires a multidisciplinary approach. High-dose corticosteroids should be started immediately based on a clinical diagnosis and steroids should not be delayed until diagnostic imaging has been performed. An initial dose of 16-mg intravenous (IV) dexamethasone followed by 4-mg dexamethasone every 4 hours provides immediate improvement in pain and possibly neurologic function. Patients should also be started on a proton pump inhibitor for gastrointestinal prophylaxis. Within 24 to 48 hours, surgery or radiation therapy (RT) should be initiated to maximize the chance of maintaining neurologic function.[6,7] A randomized trial suggested that surgery plus postoperative RT for patients with sufficient performance status and prognosis improves neurologic recovery and survival when compared to patients treated with RT alone.[8] Surgery should be strongly considered in patients with spinal instability, with compression caused by a retropulsed bone fragment, who have received RT in the same location in the past, and when histologic evaluation is needed to determine the nature of a tumor arising at an unknown primary site. Factors related to the patient (age, performance status, comorbid disease, reluctance to undergo surgery) or the disease (visceral metastases, multiple levels of spinal cord compression, presence of symptoms for more than 72 hours) may reduce the likelihood that the patient will undergo surgery. In patients greater than 65 years old, RT alone may be equally as efficacious as surgery plus postoperative RT.[9,10]

Radiation Therapy and Dose Fractionation

The optimal dose and fractionation regimen for metastatic epidural spinal cord compression is unknown and must factor in a patient's prognosis, tumor histology, efficacy, and dose tolerance of the spinal cord.

Many clinicians employ a fractionated courses of radiation to 30 Gy in 10 fractions or 20 Gy in 5 fractions with the rationale that these doses are sufficiently high to provide a good initial and durable response.[11] However, two prospective randomized studies failed to show a difference in pain control or ambulation in patients treated with 16 Gy in 2 fractions versus 30 Gy in 10 fractions or 16 Gy in 2 fractions versus a single 8 Gy dose.[12,13] Two other studies suggested no difference in improving ambulation, but some

TABLE 4.1 SINS Component and Numerical Score. A SINS Score of 0–6 Denotes Stability, 7–12 Denotes Possibly Impending, and 13–18 Denotes Instability[5]

SINS Component	Score
Location	
Junctional (occiput–C2, C7–T2, T11–L1, L5–S1)	3
Mobile spine (C3–C6, L2–L4)	2
Semirigid (T3–T10)	1
Rigid (S2–S5)	0
Pain	
Yes	3
Occasional pain but not mechanical	1
Pain-free lesion	0
Bone lesions	
Lytic	2
Mixed (lytic/blastic)	1
Blastic	0
Radiographic spinal alignment	
Subluxation/translation present	4
Kyphosis/scoliosis	2
Normal alignment	0
Vertebral body collapse	
>50% collapse	3
<50% collapse	2
No collapse with >50% body involved	1
None of the above	0
Posterolateral involvement of spinal elements	
Bilateral	3
Unilateral	1
None of the above	0

improvement in local control when longer courses are given to patients with MSCC.[14,15] While any of the studied fractionation schemes (30 Gy in 10 fractions, 16 Gy in 2 fractions, and 8 Gy in 1 fraction) are reasonable for the primary treatment of MSCC, the shorter courses may be more appropriate for those with poor overall prognoses while those with a better prognosis may have a greater benefit with longer courses of RT. The optimal dose for postoperative RT is also unknown, though 30 Gy in 10 fractions is commonly used in the United States.

The role for stereotactic body radiation therapy (SBRT) in the treatment of MSCC is unclear and currently under investigation. There are no randomized control trials demonstrating equivalence or superiority to three-dimensional (3D) conformal radiation therapy (CRT), though early results are promising. Prospective randomized data will help define the best uses of this technology.[16] Routine use should be avoided until sufficient evidence justifies the substantive increase in cost relative to standard radiation therapy. For patients who require urgent RT, the complexity of treatment planning, dependence on meticulous body immobilization, and the potential for increased side effects including myelitis, dermatitis, and vertebral compression fractures with high dose per fraction make this modality of radiation treatment challenging and less practical.[17–19] Though proton therapy has dosimetric advantages over photon radiation, it is not used for palliation of MSCC (Personal communication with Dr. Anita Mahajan).

TREATMENT PLANNING

Target Delineation

If possible, patients should undergo a CT simulation scan for treatment planning. Patients should be in a supine position with appropriate immobilization. Though many use a vac-fix, the potential need to treat adjacent areas and precisely recreate prior RT fields to minimize or eliminate overlap may argue for use of commercially available immobilization devices or a simple headrest and bolster. In addition, some patients may require prone simulation due to pain. If a recent MRI is available, the MRI should be fused with the CT simulation scan to improve target delineation. Both CT and MRI can be used to determine the depth of the vertebral surface of the cord beneath the skin surface. If a CT simulation is unavailable, fluoroscopic simulation can be performed. In this setting, the use of a wire may help to delineate the skin surface to ensure the distance to the posterior surface of vertebral bodies on a lateral radiograph.

The gross tumor volume (GTV) is best seen as the T1-enhancing abnormality or the nonenhancing tumor on T2 or fluid-attenuated inversion recovery (FLAIR) images. If there is no residual tumor after surgical resection, the GTV is defined as the resection cavity. Surrounding edema is not included in the GTV. The clinical target volume (CTV) includes the T2 and FLAIR abnormality, and clinical suspicion for microscopic disease. The width of the posterior fields should encompass the spinal canal with a 1- to 1.5-cm margin. The CTV should also include one vertebral level above and below the GTV to prevent marginal recurrence. The planning target volume (PTV) margins should account for daily variations in patient setup, and potential mass effect from cord edema.

If a patient is being treated urgently a clinical setup can be performed for the first treatment fraction. Using lateral kilovolt (kV) imaging, the depth beyond the mass can be calculated, and the patient can be treated in a source-axis distance (SAD) setup.

Treatment Techniques

Tumors in the cervical spine are often treated with opposed laterals. This technique minimizes radiation dose and consequent side effects within the oral cavity and pharyngeal structures. Tumors in the cervical-thoracic region can be treated with split beam approaches with opposed lateral fields to the upper spine, and a single posterior to anterior (PA) field for the area of the spine below with careful matching of fields. Patients with thoracic spine tumors can be treated with PA fields, opposed anterior to posterior (AP)–PA beams preferentially weighted, or opposed lateral beams. In the lumbar region, a four-field approach using AP–PA and opposed laterals can be used to reduce dose to the kidneys.

If using two-dimensional (2D) or 3D-CRT, fields should extend one vertebral body above and one vertebral body below the MSCC. This ensures that the area of concern is fully covered as isodose lines bow in at the field edges. To facilitate future treatment plans, the top of the radiation field should match the top of the vertebrae to facilitate future treatment plans, and consideration should be given to the use of a half-beam block. Treatment plans should have a reasonably homogenous dose distribution; this can be achieved by a mix of low-energy and high-energy photons and unequal beam weighting.

Laterals for MSCC of the upper cervical (C) spine
Tumors involving the upper cervical spine can be treated with opposed lateral fields to avoid unnecessary radiation to the oral cavity and hypopharynx (Figure 4.1). However, if the lesion is too inferior, then the shoulders may block the lateral fields. A PA field would be most appropriate in this case.

Single PA field thoracic (T) spine
Figure 4.2 depicts the isodose curves used to treat a 78-year-old man with metastatic prostate cancer who had bone lesions involving the thoracic (T) spine at T2 through T7 with extramedullary extension into the spinal column. A single PA beam was used to encompass the gross disease seen on

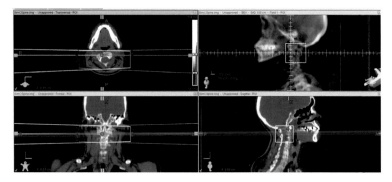

FIGURE 4.1 Opposed lateral beams for the treatment of the upper cervical spine.

the planning CT scan. The 100% isodose line encompasses the entire spinal canal. The fields extended laterally to encompass the width of the vertebral body. The sagittal view shows that the 100% isodose line extends anteriorly to encompass the spinal canal.

Single PA field lumbar (L) spine
Figure 4.3 depicts the treatment plan for a 58-year-old male with metastatic renal cell carcinoma with posterior epidural tumor invading into the cauda equina. A single 6-megavolt (MV) PA field was used to encompass the gross disease that was encroaching posteriorly through the lamina and into the vertebral foramen. The 100% isodose line covers the anterior edge of the vertebral foramen.

AP–PA treatment of the lumbar (L) spine
Tumors of the lumbar region may require opposed AP–PA fields because of the lumbar curvature and the deep location of the vertebral canal near the midline of the abdomen. Depending on the depth of coverage, a single PA field may result in high dose to the subcutaneous tissue. In Figure 4.4, a 62-year-old male with metastatic bladder cancer has metastatic disease invading into the anterior vertebral body. A parallel-opposed field was used to create a radiation treatment plan with a homogenous dose covering the disease.

Intensity-modulated or volumetric-modulated radiation therapy treatment of the entire cervical spine
Figure 4.5 depicts the treatment of a 47-year-old woman with metastatic breast cancer involving the cervical spine at C2 to C7. Since the patient's shoulders would block parallel-opposed lateral fields, an intensity-modulated RT or

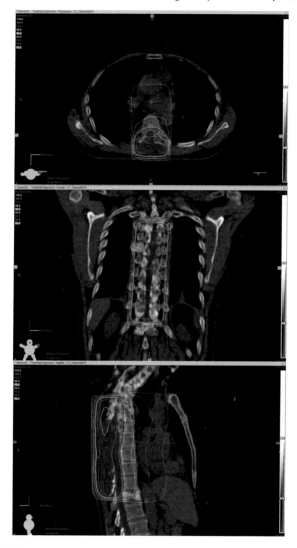

FIGURE 4.2 Axial, coronal, and sagittal images depicting the isodose lines for a single AP beam used to treat vertebral bodies T2 to T7.

volumetric-modulated arc therapy (IMRT/VMAT) plan was used to treat the spine and reduce esophagitis by limiting the exit dose. Since esophagitis typically lasts only for a few days and can be managed conservatively, a single PA field is simpler and more cost effective.

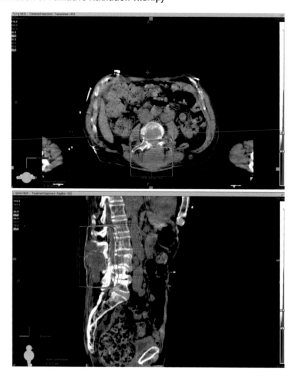

FIGURE 4.3 Axial and sagittal images depicting the isodose lines for a single PA beam used to treat the lumbar spine.

Reirradiation for infield recurrences

Advances in systemic therapy have improved overall survival with patients with metastatic cancer. As a result, radiation oncologists encounter patients with recurrent or progressive spinal metastases causing spinal cord compression. It is important to fuse previous radiation treatment fields on current planning CT scan, so as not to exceed a spinal cord dose threshold of 45 Gy. In a retrospective trial, spinal reirradiation with 8 Gy in 1 fraction, 15 Gy in 5 fractions, 20 Gy in 5 fractions, 21 Gy in 7 fractions, and 20 Gy in 10 fractions improved (25%) or stabilized (50%) motor function with no late radiation myelopathy observed. A prospective, randomized trial of reirradiation that included retreatment of the spine demonstrated that 20 Gy in 5 or 8 fractions was equivalent to 8 Gy in a single fraction for uncomplicated bone metastasis. Since 8 Gy in 1 fraction is more cost effective, noninferior, and less toxic, it is the preferred reirradiation regimen. The trial included patients treated with specific prior regimens and the inclusion criteria should be considered when reirradiating

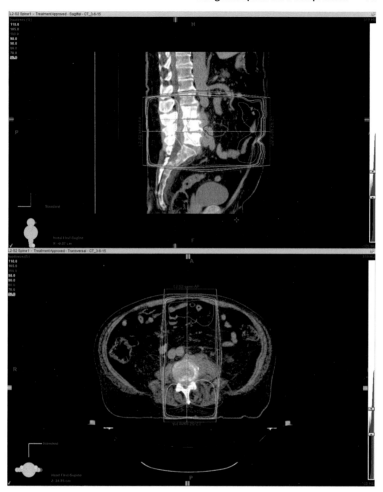

FIGURE 4.4 Sagittal and axial images depicting AP–PA treatment of the lumbar spine.

the spine. Though this trial does not directly apply to patients with spinal cord compression, it does shed light on spinal cord tolerance to radiation.[20] Reirradiation was safe and effective when the cumulative biological effective dose (BED) was less than 120 Gy (alpha/beta of 2).[21] SBRT as a primary treatment for metastatic epidural spinal cord compression is feasible but there is a lack of long-term outcomes compared to surgical intervention and/or external beam radiation therapy.[22]

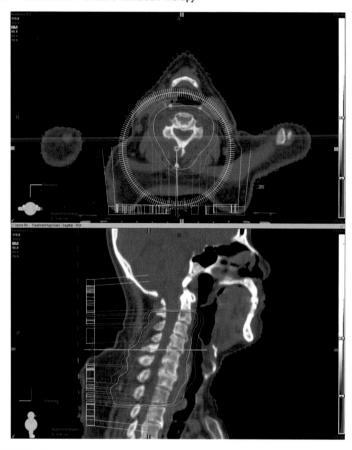

FIGURE 4.5 Axial and sagittal images of a single VMAT arc plan to treat vertebral bodies C2 to C7.

Follow-Up

After completion of RT, follow-up is important in order to assess for changes in pain, motor function, and sensation. There are no studies or guidelines addressing follow-up of treatment for MSCC. However, if pain has not improved within 2 weeks, the physician will need to prescribe or increase steroids, try other classes of analgesics, or reevaluate for concern for disease progression with new radiologic imaging.

Acute and Late Effects

Acute side effects include dermatitis, pain flare, and nausea. The most common acute effect is grade 1 to 2 dermatitis over the treated area. Patients can use petroleum-based products to minimize dryness and erythema. Additionally, pain flare along the spinal cord typically occurs within 1 to 4 days after radiotherapy. Prophylactic use of 8-mg dexamethasone has been shown to reduce episodes of pain flare by 8% compared to placebo.[23] Lastly, patients may experience nausea and diarrhea from low-dose radiation in the intestine. Antiemetics, such as 8 mg of ondansetron, are given prior to the dose of radiation to prevent or reduce the development of radiation-induced nausea when the stomach or intestines are in the radiation fields.

In 2 to 6 months, the patient may develop a reversible myelopathy secondary to transient demyelination characterized by shock-like radiation sensations to extremities when the neck is flexed (L'Hermitte's sign). Symptoms are self-limiting and no therapy is required. If symptomatic, a trial of glucocorticoids can be prescribed. If the patient does not respond, care must be taken to taper off the glucocorticoids since chronic steroid use can result in steroid myopathy.

Rarely, chronic progressive myelopathy is a late complication of radiation that is progressive and chronic with no treatment available. Tumor progression may also cause myelitis and retreatment can be considered, taking into account the spinal cord or cauda equina tolerance and prior delivered dose.[24] In pediatric patients, the risk of a secondary neoplasia, spine deformity, and height loss following radiation is significant. Treatment plans should generally include the entire vertebral body to reduce asymmetric growth.

CLINICAL PEARLS

- High-dose corticosteroids should be started immediately based on a clinical diagnosis of MSCC.
- Shorter courses of radiation (16 Gy in 2 fractions and 8 Gy in 1 fraction) may be more appropriate for those with poor overall prognoses, while those with better prognoses may have greater durable responses with longer courses of RT (30 Gy in 10 fractions).
- The SINS classification system can be used as a guideline regarding the appropriate point to request neurosurgical referral.
- Opposed lateral fields or PA-only fields can be used instead of AP–PA to limit toxicity to nearby normal tissues anterior to the region being treated

SELF-ASSESSMENT

Questions

1. True/False: A patient with pain due to spinal cord compression at vertebral level C7 with bilateral involvement of the spinal elements should be referred for surgical evaluation?

2. Which dose regimen is preferred in patients with spinal cord compression and a Karnofsky performance score (KPS) of 50?
   A. 35 Gy in 14 fractions
   B. 30 Gy in 10 fractions
   C. 20 Gy in 5 fractions
   D. 8 Gy in 1 fraction

3. Which beam arrangement is preferred when treating the lower cervical spine?
   A. Opposed laterals
   B. AP–PA
   C. Single PA beam
   D. Single AP beam

Answers

1. True. This patient has a spinal instability neoplastic score (SINS) score of 9 due to a junctional location (three points), the presence of pain (three points), and bilateral involvement of the spinal elements (3 points). Patients with SINS score greater than 7 should have surgical evaluation for possible spinal instability.

2. Answer D. Randomized data have demonstrated equivalence (in terms of pain control and ambulation) of 16 Gy in 2 fractions or 8 Gy in a single fraction for patients with Eastern Cooperative Oncology Group (ECOG) ≥ 2 (KPS ≤ 70). For patients with limited life expectancies, the shortest course of radiation therapy to provide a therapeutic effect is preferred.

3. Answer C. When treating the lower cervical spine, a single PA beam is generally preferred. The shoulders typically interfere with lateral beams and AP–PA treatment delivers more dose to the oropharynx and esophagus. Shorter courses of radiation therapy (8 Gy in 1 fraction) cause little to no esophagitis; depending on the planned dose, AP–PA may be acceptable. In patients with a longer life expectancy, longer courses of radiation therapy (30 Gy in 10 fractions) have been associated with improved local control. For these patients, a single PA field is preferred. IMRT or VMAT can be used but are more complicated and expensive.

REFERENCES

1. Rades D, Dunst J, Schild SE. The first score predicting overall survival in patients with metastatic spinal cord compression. *Cancer*. January 1, 2008;112(1):157-161. PubMed PMID: 17948910.

2. Bayley A, Milosevic M, Blend R, et al. A prospective study of factors predicting clinically occult spinal cord compression in patients with metastatic prostate carcinoma. *Cancer*. July 15, 2001;92(2):303-310. PubMed PMID: 11466683.

3. Bilsky MH, Lis E, Raizer J, et al. The diagnosis and treatment of metastatic spinal tumor. *Oncologist.* 1999;4(6):459-469. PubMed PMID: 10631690.

4. Shah LM, Salzman KL. Imaging of spinal metastatic disease. *Int J Surg Oncol.* 2011;2011:769753. PubMed PMID: 22312523. Pubmed Central PMCID: PMC3263660.

5. Fourney DR, Frangou EM, Ryken TC, et al. Spinal instability neoplastic score: an analysis of reliability and validity from the spine oncology study group. *J Clin Oncol.* August 1, 2011;29(22):3072-3077. PubMed PMID: 21709187.

6. Greenberg HS, Kim JH, Posner JB. Epidural spinal cord compression from metastatic tumor: results with a new treatment protocol. *Ann Neurol.* 1980;8(4):361-366.

7. Prasad D, Schiff D. Malignant spinal-cord compression. *Lancet Oncol.* January 2005;6(1):15-24. PubMed PMID: 15629272. Epub 2005/01/05. eng.

8. Patchell RA, Tibbs PA, Regine WF, et al. Direct decompressive surgical resection in the treatment of spinal cord compression caused by metastatic cancer: a randomised trial. *Lancet.* August 20–26, 2005;366(9486):643-648. PubMed PMID: 16112300.

9. Chi JH, Gokaslan Z, McCormick P, et al. Selecting treatment for patients with malignant epidural spinal cord compression-does age matter?: results from a randomized clinical trial. *Spine (Phila Pa 1976).* March 1, 2009;34(5): 431-435. PubMed PMID: 19212272.

10. Rades D, Huttenlocher S, Dunst J, et al. Matched pair analysis comparing surgery followed by radiotherapy and radiotherapy alone for metastatic spinal cord compression. *J Clin Oncol.* August 1, 2010;28(22):3597-3604. PubMed PMID: 20606090.

11. Loblaw DA, Perry J, Chambers A, Laperriere NJ. Systematic review of the diagnosis and management of malignant extradural spinal cord compression: the Cancer Care Ontario Practice Guidelines Initiative's Neuro-Oncology Disease Site Group. *J Clin Oncol.* March 20, 2005;23(9):2028-2037. PubMed PMID: 15774794.

12. Maranzano E, Bellavita R, Rossi R, et al. Short-course versus split-course radiotherapy in metastatic spinal cord compression: results of a phase III, randomized, multicenter trial. *J Clin Oncol.* May 20, 2005;23(15):3358-3365. PubMed PMID: 15738534.

13. Maranzano E, Trippa F, Casale M, et al. 8 Gy single-dose radiotherapy is effective in metastatic spinal cord compression: results of a phase III randomized multicentre Italian trial. *Radiother Oncol.* November 2009;93(2): 174-179. PubMed PMID: 19520448.

14. Rades D, Fehlauer F, Stalpers LJ, et al. A prospective evaluation of two radiotherapy schedules with 10 versus 20 fractions for the treatment of metastatic

spinal cord compression: final results of a multicenter study. *Cancer.* December 1, 2004;101(11):2687-2692. PubMed PMID: 15493037.

15. Rades D, Stalpers LJ, Veninga T, et al. Evaluation of five radiation schedules and prognostic factors for metastatic spinal cord compression. *J Clin Oncol.* May 20, 2005;23(15):3366-3375. PubMed PMID: 15908648.

16. RTOG. RTOG 0631: A Phase II/III Study of Image-Guided Radiosurgery/ SBRT for Localized Spine Metastasis—RTOG CCOP Study 2006 [January 31 2016]. Available at https://www.rtog.org/ClinicalTrials/Protocol Table/StudyDetails.aspx?study=0631.

17. Gibbs IC, Patil C, Gerszten PC, et al. Delayed radiation-induced myelopathy after spinal radiosurgery. *Neurosurgery.* February 2009;64(2 suppl):A67-A72. PubMed PMID: 19165076.

18. Ryu S, Jin JY, Jin R, et al. Partial volume tolerance of the spinal cord and complications of single-dose radiosurgery. *Cancer.* February 1, 2007;109(3): 628-636. PubMed PMID: 17167762.

19. Chang EL, Shiu AS, Mendel E, et al. Phase I/II study of stereotactic body radiotherapy for spinal metastasis and its pattern of failure. *J Neurosurg Spine.* August 2007;7(2):151-160. PubMed PMID: 17688054.

20. Chow E, van der Linden YM, Roos D, et al. Single versus multiple fractions of repeat radiation for painful bone metastases: a randomised, controlled, non-inferiority trial. *Lancet Oncol.* February 2014;15(2):164-171. PubMed PMID: 24369114.

21. Rades D, Stalpers LJ, Veninga T, Hoskin PJ. Spinal reirradiation after short-course RT for metastatic spinal cord compression. *Int J Radiat Oncol Biol Phys.* November 1, 2005;63(3):872-875. PubMed PMID: 15939549.

22. Ryu S, Rock J, Jain R, et al. Radiosurgical decompression of metastatic epidural compression. *Cancer.* May 1, 2010;116(9):2250-2257. PubMed PMID: 20209611.

23. Chow E, Meyer RM, Ding K, et al. Prophylactic dexamethasone for radiation-induced bone-pain flare—Authors' reply. *Lancet Oncol.* February 2016;17(2):e40-e41. PubMed PMID: 26868346.

24. Nieder C, Grosu AL, Andratschke NH, Molls M. Update of human spinal cord reirradiation tolerance based on additional data from 38 patients. *Int J Radiat Oncol Biol Phys*. December 1, 2006;66(5):1446-1449. PubMed PMID: 17084560.

5   Brain Metastases

Mohammad Hasan and May N. Tsao

INTRODUCTION

Demographics

Metastatic disease to the brain is the most common intracranial tumor.[1] The incidence of brain metastases is at least 10% for patients diagnosed with lung cancer, renal cancer, colorectal cancer, breast cancer, and melanoma,[2] with the highest incidence being 20% for lung cancer. With an aging population it is expected that the number of patients with metastatic disease will increase, including the number of patients with metastatic disease to the brain.

Prognosis

From a clinical standpoint, survival estimates for patients with brain metastases are important for patients and families to help guide health care decisions and may provide the impetus for patients to focus on work and personal (including social and financial) planning. From a research perspective, survival comparisons in trials for patients with brain metastases depend not only on the intervention but also on prognostic factors. Outcomes comparing interventions for patients with brain metastases are only valid when the trial arms are balanced with known and unknown prognostic factors.

The Radiation Therapy Oncology Group recursive partitioning analysis (RTOG RPA)[3] examined statistically significant prognostic factors for survival for newly diagnosed patients treated in three RTOG whole brain radiation therapy (WBRT) trials, examining different dose fractionation schemes alone or with radiosensitizers. Published in 1997, the RTOG RPA consisted of three classes. Class I patients were patients with Karnofsky performance score (KPS) over 70, whose age were less than 65, and with a controlled primary and the brain as the only sites of visible cancer. RPA Class I patients had a median survival of 7.1 months. Class III RTOG RPA patients were those with a KPS less than 70. These patients had a median survival of 2.1 months. Class II RTOG RPA patients were brain metastases patients who do not meet the criteria for either Class I or Class III categories. Their median survival was 4.2 months.

However, the recognition that other prognostic factors (such as histology and number of brain metastases) were not captured in the RTOG RPA emerged. In 2010, the diagnosis specific graded prognostic assessment (DS-GPA) was published.[4] Characteristics from a retrospective database of 5,067 patients with newly diagnosed brain metastases from 11 institutions treated between 1985 and 2007 were analyzed. Unlike the RTOG RPA, the DS-GPA depends on histology. A score is given for each significant prognostic factor. Survival estimates were obtained based on the sum of scores given a specific histology (Tables 5.1 and 5.2).

In 2012, a further refinement in prognosis for breast cancer metastases to the brain was made based on a multi-institutional retrospective database of 400 breast cancer patients[5] treated for newly diagnosed brain metastases (Tables 5.3 and 5.4).

TABLE 5.1 Graded Prognostic Factor Scoring Table[4]

	GPA Scoring Criteria		
	0	**0.5**	**1**
	Small Cell and Non–Small Cell Lung Cancer		
Age	>60	50–59	<50
Number of brain metastases	>3	2–3	1
KPS	<70	70–80	90–100
Extracranial metastases	Present	–	Absent
	GPA Scoring Criteria		
	0	**1**	**2**
	Renal Cell Cancer and Melanoma		
KPS	<70	70–80	90–100
Number of brain metastases	>3	2–3	1

	GPA Scoring Criteria				
	0	**1**	**2**	**3**	**4**
	Breast Cancer and GI Cancer				
KPS	<70	70	80	90	100

GI, gastrointestinal; GPA, graded prognostic assessment; KPS, Karnofsky performance score.

TABLE 5.2 Median Survival (in Months) Based on Overall GPA Score[4]

DS-GPA	Breast Cancer	NSCLC	SCLC	GI	RCC	Melanoma
0–1	6.1	3	2.8	3.1	3.3	3.4
1.5–2.5	9.4	6.5	5.3	4.4	7.3	4.7
3	16.9	11.3	9.6	6.9	11.3	8.8
3.5–4	18.7	14.8	17.1	13.5	14.8	13.2

DS-GPA, diagnosis-specific graded prognostic assessment; GI, gastrointestinal; NSCLC, non–small-cell lung cancer; RCC, renal cell cancer; SCLC, small cell lung cancer.

TABLE 5.3 Graded Prognostic Index for Breast Cancer Brain Metastases[5]

	GPA Scoring Criteria				
	0	0.5	1	1.5	2
KPS	≤50	60	70–80	90–100	–
Genetic	Basal	–	Luminal A	HER2	Luminal B
Age (years)	≥60	<60	–	–	–

GPA, graded prognostic assessment; KPS, Karnofsky performance score.

TABLE 5.4 Median Survival in Months for Breast Graded Prognostic Assessment[5]

Breast-GPA	Median Survival (Months)
0–1	3.4
1.5–2	7.7
2.5–3	15.1
3.5–4	25.3

GPA, graded prognostic assessment.

MANAGEMENT

Steroids

Steroids provide temporary relief of symptoms due to intracerebral edema from brain metastases. The steroid of choice is dexamethasone and the starting dose of 4 to 8 mg per day has been suggested in clinical practice guidelines.[6] However, if a patient experiences severe symptoms of increased intracranial pressure, higher doses such as 16 mg per day or more should be considered.

The only contemporary randomized trial that has examined the use of optimal supportive care versus optimal supportive care and WBRT was the QUARTZ trial.[7,8] An interim analysis (reporting on 151 patients out of a planned 534 patients) indicated no detriment in quality of life, overall survival, or quality-adjusted life years (QALYs) between the two arms.[7] In this interim analysis,

8% (12/151), 42% (64/151), and 50% (75/151) were classified as RTOG RPA classes I, II, and III, respectively. Overall survival between the two arms was similar for 49 days for optimal supportive care and WBRT versus 51 days for optimal supportive care alone (hazard ratio [HR] 1.11, 95% CI 0.80–1.53). The final trial results have been published in abstract form.[7] For the 538 patients recruited, there was no significant difference in overall survival [HR 1.05 (95% CI 0.89–1.26)]. The median survival of optimal supportive care and WBRT versus optimal supportive care alone was 65 versus 57 days, respectively. Overall quality of life or steroid use was no different between the two arms.

An older trial[9] randomized patients to prednisone with or without WBRT. The proportion of patients with improved performance status was similar between the two arms and median survival was 10 weeks in the steroid alone arm versus 14 weeks in the combined arm (*P* value not stated). The increase in median survival in the WBRT and prednisone arm is most likely attributed to the efficacy of radiation therapy in delaying the growth of brain metastases.

As such, there are subsets of brain metastases patients who have poor prognoses (such as patients with poor performance status and progressive extracranial disease despite systemic therapy) who are unlikely to benefit from radiotherapeutic intervention.

Single Brain Metastasis

The benefit of surgery for the management of selected patients with resectable single brain metastasis emerged from randomized trials published in the 1980s and 1990s (Table 5.5a–d). Randomized trials support the use of surgery to improve survival as compared to WBRT alone in selected patients with controlled systemic disease and a resectable single brain metastasis.[10] The histologies excluded in the trials on the use of surgery were radiosensitive histologies such as small cell lung cancer, lymphoma, leukemia, and germ cell tumors. The use of postoperative WBRT for patients with resected brain metastases improves overall brain control but does not improve survival.[11]

TABLE 5.5 Randomized Trials for Single Brain Metastasis

(a) Surgery for Single Brain Metastasis (WBRT and Surgery vs. WBRT)

	Interventions	Overall Survival (Median)	Duration of Functional Independence
Patchell et al.[12]	WBRT and surgery vs. WBRT	40 wk vs. 15 wk (*P* <.01)	38 wk vs. 8 wk (*P* <.005)

(*continued*)

TABLE 5.5 Randomized Trials for Single Brain Metastasis (*continued*)

(a) Surgery for Single Brain Metastasis (WBRT and Surgery vs. WBRT)

	Interventions	Overall Survival (Median)	Duration of Functional Independence
Noordijk et al.[13]	WBRT and surgery vs. WBRT	10 mo vs. 6 mo (*P* = .04)	–
Mintz et al.[14]	WBRT and surgery vs. WBRT	5.6 mo vs. 6.3 mo (*P* = .24)	–

WBRT, whole brain radiation therapy.

(b) Surgery Versus Surgery and WBRT for Single Brain Metastasis

	Interventions	Overall Survival	Overall Brain Control	Treated Lesion Control/New Brain Sites Control	Percentage Single Brain Metastasis
Patchell et al.[15]	Surgery vs. Surgery and WBRT (All patients with single brain metastasis)	43 wk vs. 48 wk (*P* = .39)	30% vs. 82% (*P* < .001)	54%/63% vs. 90%/86% (*P* < 0.001/ *P* < 0.01)	100%
Kocher et al.[16]	Surgery (or SRS) vs. Surgery (or SRS) and WBRT (45% of patients in the trial had single brain metastasis)	10.7 mo vs. 10.9 mo (*P* = .89)*	22% vs. 52% (*P* < .01)*	41%/58% vs. 73%/77% (*P* < .001/ *P* = .023)**	45%

SRS, stereotactic radiosurgery; WBRT, whole brain radiation therapy.
*Includes single and multiple brain metastases treated with SRS or surgery.
**Includes single and multiple brain metastases treated with surgery.

(*continued*)

TABLE 5.5 Randomized Trials for Single Brain Metastasis (*continued*)

(c) Radiosurgery for Single Brain Metastasis (WBRT and SRS vs. WBRT)

	Interventions	Proportion of Patients in the Trial With Single Brain Metastasis	Overall Survival	Overall Brain Control	Treated Lesion Control/ New Brain Sites Control
Andrews et al.[17]	WBRT and SRS vs. WBRT	56%	6.5 mo vs. 4.9 mo (P = .0393)	75% vs. 70% (P = .13) At 1 y*	82%/NR vs. 71%/NR (P = .01) At 1 y*

NR, not reported; SRS, stereotactic radiosurgery; WBRT, whole brain radiation therapy.
*Includes single and multiple brain metastases.

(d) Radiosurgery for Single Brain Metastasis (SRS vs. WBRT and SRS)

	Interventions	Proportion of Patients in the Trial With Single Brain Metastasis	Overall Survival	Overall Brain Control	Treated Lesion Control/New Brain Sites Control
Kocher et al.[16]	SRS (or surgery) vs. SRS (or surgery) and WBRT	67%	10.7 mo vs. 10.9 mo (P = .89)*	22% vs. 52% (P <.01)*	69%/52% vs. 81%/67% (P = .04/ P = .023)** At 2 y
Aoyama et al.[18]	SRS vs. WBRT and SRS	66%	8 mo vs. 7.5 mo (P = .42)***	24% vs. 53% (P < .001) At 1 y***	73%/36% vs. 89%/59% (P = .002/ P = .03) At 1 y***

(*continued*)

TABLE 5.5 Randomized Trials for Single Brain Metastasis (*continued*)

(d) Radiosurgery for Single Brain Metastasis (SRS vs. WBRT and SRS)

	Interventions	Proportion of Patients in the Trial With Single Brain Metastasis	Overall Survival	Overall Brain Control	Treated Lesion Control/New Brain Sites Control
Chang et al.[19]	SRS vs. WBRT and SRS	57%	15.2 mo vs. 5.7 mo (*P* = .003)	27% vs. 73% (*P* = .0003) At 1 y	67%/45% vs. 100%/73% (*P* = .012/ *P* = .02) At 1 y***

SRS, stereotactic radiosurgery; WBRT, whole brain radiation therapy.
*Includes single and multiple brain metastases treated with SRS or surgery.
**Includes single and multiple brain metastases treated with SRS.
***Includes single and multiple brain metastases.

In a meta-analysis of three randomized trials on resection and WBRT versus WBRT alone for single brain metastasis,[20] no significant difference in survival was noted, HR 0.74 (95% confidence interval [CI] 0.39–1.40, *P* = .35). However, there was a high degree of heterogeneity between trials. In particular, the Mintz et al. trial[14] included a higher percentage of patients with active extracranial disease. One trial[12] reported that surgery and WBRT increased the duration of functionally independent survival (FIS) HR 0.42 (95% CI 0.22–0.80, *P* <.008). There is a trend for surgery and WBRT to reduce the number of deaths due to neurological cause odds ratio (OR) 0.57 (95% CI 0.29–1.10, *P* = .09).

However, the use of WBRT has been shown to negatively affect neurocognition and quality of life.[19,21] For small (<4 cm) single brain metastasis, particularly those located in eloquent areas not resectable, radiosurgery alone is currently being used to control the targeted metastasis and to avoid the side effects of WBRT. In addition, experimental strategies (e.g., surgery for single brain metastasis followed by postoperative cavity radiosurgery or focal postoperative cavity radiation) to avoid WBRT have emerged.

Four or Less Brain Metastases

The use of radiosurgery alone versus radiosurgery and WBRT has been studied in numerous randomized trials.[16,18,19,21] These trials included good performance status patients with 1 to 4 brain metastases less than 4 cm in size and inactive extra-cranial disease. Overall there is improved whole brain control with the use of adjuvant WBRT added to radiosurgery. In all but one trial,[19] overall survival is not different with the use of radiosurgery and WBRT as compared to radiosurgery alone. Two trials[19,21] reported worsening in neurocognitive function at 3 to 4 months after adjuvant WBRT as compared to radiosurgery alone.

In 2014, the American Society for Radiation Oncology's (ASTRO) "Choosing Wisely" campaign recommended against the routine use of adjuvant WBRT with stereotactic radiosurgery (SRS) for patients with a limited number of brain metastases. Randomized trials do not demonstrate a survival benefit in this setting. WBRT is associated with diminished cognitive function, worse quality of life, and more fatigue. Patients treated with SRS alone can be surveilled for the development of metastases in the brain. Adjuvant WBRT can be carefully considered at the time of recurrence to promote the best quality of life.[1]

Patients who are ineligible for radiosurgery, due to the size of the metastatic deposits, poor performance status, and/or active extra-cranial disease may be treated with WBRT and/or supportive care.

Five or More Brain Metastases

Controversy exists as to whether patients with 5 to 10 brain metastases (all <4 cm in size) should be treated with WBRT or SRS alone. Proponents for SRS alone advocate that in the absence of survival advantage as compared to WBRT, patients should undergo SRS alone as there may be neurocognitive and quality of life sparing with the avoidance of WBRT.[22] On the other hand, justification for the use of WBRT includes improved overall brain control as compared to SRS alone. Patients treated with SRS alone are at much higher risk of distant brain relapse which also is associated with neurocognitive decline.[23] In terms of expense and resources, SRS is more costly and resource intensive to administer compared to WBRT.

At present, there are no published phase III randomized controlled trials which directly compare SRS alone versus WBRT for patients with five or more brain metastases. Outcomes of interest include survival, treated brain metastases control, overall brain control, quality of life, and neurocognition.

EMERGING THERAPIES

Neurocognitive Protection

Experimental strategies such as hippocampal radiation sparing,[24] and the use of medications such as memantine[25] and donepezil,[26] have been used with the intent to spare neurocognitive function with WBRT.

Hippocampal Sparing

Neural stem cells in the subgranular zone of the hippocampus are believed to play a role in replenishing depleted neurons. It is believed that WBRT adversely affects neurocognition by depleting neural stem cells in the subgranular zone of the hippocampus. The hippocampus is rarely the site of brain metastases and as a result efforts to spare the hippocampus and thereby possibly spare memory decline with WBRT were undertaken.[24]

In the RTOG-0933 phase II trial, the authors reported that the use of hippocampal sparing WBRT was associated with preservation of memory and quality of life as compared to historical series of patients.[27]

Pharmacological Intervention for Neurocognition

A randomized double-blind, placebo-controlled trial reported that memantine was well tolerated and had similar toxicity to placebo in patients treated with WBRT. Overall, patients treated with memantine had better delayed time to cognitive decline and reduced rate of decline in memory, executive function, and processing speed as compared to placebo.[25]

Another phase III randomized placebo-controlled trial examined the use of donepezil in patients treated with partial or WBRT. While donepezil did not improve overall composite cognitive scores, it did result in some improvement with respect to several cognitive functions, particularly among patients with greater baseline impairments.[26]

Molecular Agents

Over the past decade, targeted agents which inhibit specific molecular targets in cancer cells have been developed. The classification of targeted therapies for cancer includes tyrosine kinase inhibitors, monoclonal antibodies, and cancer vaccines.[28] Brain metastases have shown responses to some targeted agents.

Lung cancer
A randomized phase III trial of WBRT and radiosurgery versus radiosurgery alone with either temozolomide or erlotinib (an epidermal growth factor receptor inhibitor) was reported for 126 out of 381 planned patients.[29] This trial closed early due to poor accrual. The median survival times were worse for the WBRT and radiosurgery with temozolomide or erlotinib as compared to WBRT and radiosurgery alone (6.3 vs. 6.1 months vs. 13.4 months, respectively), although the differences did not reach statistical significance likely due to the small numbers. The addition of temozolomide or erlotinib was associated with more frequent grades 3 to 5 toxicity as compared to WBRT and

radiosurgery alone (41%, 49%, vs. 11%, respectively). Lack of tumor EGFR testing was a major limitation of this trial.

A few small prospective and retrospective series report brain metastases response with the use of EGFR targeted agents alone, without brain radiation.[30–32]

Breast cancer

The LANDSCAPE prospective multi-institutional phase II trial[33] enrolled 45 HER2 positive breast cancer patients with brain metastases (who did not receive prior WBRT) to lapatinib (a tyrosine kinase inhibitor) and capecitabine. Intracranial response (all partial) was seen in 65.9% of patients. However, 49% had grade 3 or 4 toxicity. No grade 5 toxicities were noted.

Other studies have also supported the finding of intracranial response to lapatinib alone.[34] In a multicenter phase II trial of lapatinib for salvage of 242 previously treated brain metastases patients with HER2-positive breast cancer, 6% experienced 50% or more volumetric reduction in brain metastases, 21% showed 20% or more volume reduction in brain metastases.

Melanoma

In a multi-institutional phase II trial, dabrafenib (a BRAF inhibitor) was associated with 39.3% intracranial response in those patients who had no prior brain therapy and 30.8% brain response in those patients who had progressive metastases after previous brain therapy.[35]

A few studies have also examined the use of vemurafenib (a BRAF inhibitor) alone in the treatment of brain metastases from melanoma and intracranial response varies from 37% to 50%.[36,37]

Ipilimumab blocks cytotoxic T-lymphocyte-associated antigen 4 (CTLA-4) and has been used experimentally either alone or with radiosurgery in a small number of patients with metastatic melanoma to the brain.[38,39]

Molecular targeted agents have not been used routinely for the initial management of newly diagnosed brain metastases patients. The targeted therapy studies have focused largely on brain responses. Further research in this modality is needed to ascertain whether there is any survival, quality of life, or symptom control benefit with these agents as compared to WBRT and/or radiosurgery.

Radiation Treatment Planning

Whole brain radiation therapy

For WBRT, the CT simulation involves the patient lying supine with the head in a neutral position by a thermoplastic mask and neck rest. The beam arrangement is lateral opposing fields with collimation to shape the beam. Shielding is used to exclude the lens and extra-cranial contents from direct irradiation. The typical fractionations used are hypofractionated regimens such as 20 Gy in 5-daily fractions or 30 Gy in 10-daily fractions. No other WBRT dose fractionation schedule has been found to result in better survival.[40]

The WBRT fractionation schedules studied in phase III randomized trials include 10 Gy in 1 fraction, 12 Gy in 2-daily fractions, 32 Gy in 20 fractions twice daily with a 22.4 Gy in 14-daily fractions boost to visible brain metastases, 40 Gy in 20 fractions twice daily, and 50 Gy in 20-daily fractions. All these different fractionation schemes were compared to either standard 30 Gy in 10-daily fractions or standard 20 Gy in 5-daily fractions. Forty percent of patients treated with a single 10 Gy to the whole brain developed acute complications (headache, nausea, vomiting, neurologic deficit, or decline in level of consciousness) compared to 27% treated to 30 Gy in 10-daily fractions. Due to the lack of formal neurocognitive testing in these trials, it is unclear which WBRT regimen, if any, might be associated with less neurocognitive decline. There is also no evidence of better symptoms or quality of life outcomes with these different WBRT fractionation schemes as compared to 20 Gy in 5-daily fractions or 30 Gy in 10-daily fractions.

The WBRT dose fractionation is prescribed at the International Commission of Radiation Units and Measurements (ICRU) reference point for radiation plans using dosimetry. Without dosimetric plans, the WBRT dose can be prescribed to midplane. Figure 5.1 demonstrates a WBRT plan in the axial and sagittal planes for a dose of 20 Gy in 5 fractions. Figure 5.2 demonstrates the radiation isodose curves and digitally reconstructed radiographs (DRRs) demonstrating field definition for a patient treated with 30 Gy in 10 fractions. A scalp block has been added using a field-in-field technique to minimize the high-dose region in the scalp, which allows more complete hair regrowth.

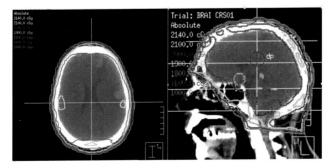

FIGURE 5.1 Axial and sagittal isodose lines for a radiation plan delivering 20 Gy in 5 fractions.

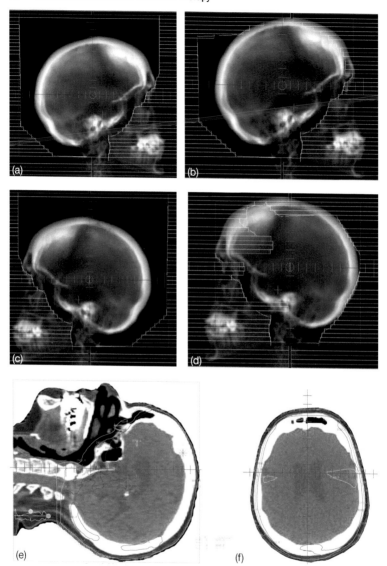

FIGURE 5.2 DRRs for the opposed laterals (a, c) and the field-in-field (b, d) beams together with sagittal (e) and axial (f) image planes with the radiation isodose curves. Dose delivered 30 Gy in 10 fractions.

Stereotactic radiosurgery

The American Association of Neurological Surgeons (AANS), the Congress of Neurological Surgeons (CNS), and the ASTRO defined SRS in 2009 to include the following criteria:

- Use of ionizing radiation to ablate target(s) in the head or spine without surgery
- High-resolution stereotactic imaging for target localization
- Multidisciplinary team participation (a neurosurgeon, radiation oncologist, and medical physicist)
- Delivery of radiation in a single or limited number of sessions (up to 5) with stereotactic immobilization that may incorporate robotics or real time imaging

All the randomized trials on SRS for brain metastases used traditional single fraction SRS methods. Specifically, a rigidly attached stereotactic frame using pins secured to the patient's skull, a stereotactic image-guidance system, and either a linear accelerator-based radiosurgery or multisource Cobalt 60 unit (Gamma Knife) were used.

Certain treatment units are also capable of delivering SRS without a frame. SRS fractionation schemes are not uniform; however, they range from 1 to 5 fractions. The doses for single fraction SRS range from typically 15 to 24 Gy, depending on the target size or volume and proximity to organs at risk. The optimal fractionated stereotactic regimen for metastatic disease to brain has yet to be determined.

The organs at risk that are typically contoured for brain metastases SRS include the lenses. Depending on the proximity of the target to organs at risk, other contours for dose constraints such as the optic nerves, chiasm, and brainstem are also of interest. Figure 5.3 demonstrates the localization of a single brain metastasis along with the 100% isodose curve for SRS. Figure 5.4 demonstrates the SRS treatment of a larger target volume and the treatment response to SRS by MRI.

Toxicity

Whole brain radiation therapy

Acute

Acute side effects of WRBRT include generalized fatigue, risk of increased intracranial pressure requiring dexamethasone use, and epilation of scalp hair. The severity and duration of fatigue are variable and multifactorial.

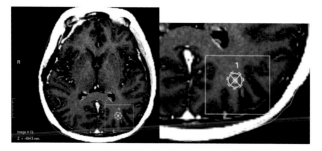

FIGURE 5.3 Stereotactic localization of a single brain metastasis in the axial plane. The yellow cross represents the isocenter. The blue line is the gross tumor volume (GTV) and the red line is the prescription isodose line, in this case 24 Gy due to the small GTV size.

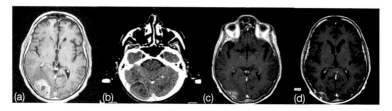

FIGURE 5.4 A patient with a target volume of 38.45 mL treated with 18 Gy. (a) Pre-SRS T1 MRI with gadolinium demonstrating the contrast-enhancing lesion in the right occipital region. (b) Treatment planning CT showing radiation dose coverage of tumor. (c) Follow-up T1 MRI with gadolinium 2 months after treatment showing significant reduction in tumor size effect. (d) Follow-up T1 MRI with gadolinium 1 year after treatment showing continued shrinkage of metastasis. Courtesy of Jared Robbins, MD.

Late

The main late side effect of WBRT is neurocognitive decline. One trial[19] reported that patients treated with the addition of WBRT to SRS were at greater risk of decline in learning and memory at 4 months compared to patients treated with SRS alone. Another trial reported in abstract form[21] reported decline in immediate recall, memory, and verbal fluency in patients treated with the addition of WBRT to SRS.

Stereotactic radiosurgery

Acute

Possible acute side effects of SRS include seizures, acute edema requiring dexamethasone use, and a small risk of infection and permanent numbness at the SRS pin sites.

Late

The risk of symptomatic radiation necrosis with SRS ranges from 2% to approximately 30% in the literature.[41]

Symptom Management

Symptomatic brain edema

Dexamethasone is the steroid of choice (due to its minimal mineralocorticoid effect and long half-life) for the management of symptomatic brain edema from brain metastases and from radiation treatment. Clinical practice guidelines recommend a starting dose of 4 to 8 mg/day for symptomatic brain edema. However, if patients have severe brain edema symptoms, higher doses such as 16 mg/day or more should be considered.[6]

Seizures

Prophylactic antiepileptic medications are not recommended in brain tumor patients as use of antiseizure medications do not significantly lower seizure incidence as compared to patients not using antiseizure medications.[42] There is a risk of adverse side effects with the use of antiepileptics.

However, antiepileptic medications should be given in the treatment for established seizures. Nonenzyme inducing antiseizure medication with less drug interactions and side effects such as levetiracetam are preferred.

SUMMARY

The management of newly diagnosed brain metastases has evolved over the decades. Treatment includes symptom management, such as the use of steroids to alleviate symptoms of brain edema. Depending on prognostic factors and the extent of brain metastases (number and volume), therapies supported by randomized trials include best supportive care, surgery, WBRT, and SRS given alone or in combination. For selected patients, SRS alone (withholding WBRT) spares neurocognition.

CLINICAL PEARLS

- Confirm the diagnosis of brain metastases. Supporting evidence includes neuroradiologic confirmation and pathologic evidence of a primary cancer. Do not get fooled by potential masqueraders of brain metastases, which are rare but important to recognize.
- The characteristics of the patient (e.g., performance status), tumor (e.g., number and size of brain metastases, extracranial disease

(*continued*)

(*continued*)
burden and activity), and treatment factors (e.g., availability of neurosurgery and SRS) will help guide treatment. Patients with poor prognoses may be best managed with dexamethasone and supportive care.

■ It is important to recognize whether certain systemic therapies should be held or not be given concurrently with brain radiation.

■ The dose, frequency, and duration of dexamethasone should be individualized based on the patient symptoms of brain edema, with the goal to minimize dexamethasone, if tolerated.

■ Antiseizure medications are prescribed for the treatment of seizures and are not routinely given for prophylaxis.

SELF-ASSESSMENT

Question

1. A 65-year-old male patient with metastatic colon cancer to liver and brain is referred to have radiation to the brain. His KPS is 80. A volumetric thin slice MRI with gadolinium shows a 1.8-cm metastasis in his left temporal lobe. What options are available to this patient? What is his median overall survival?

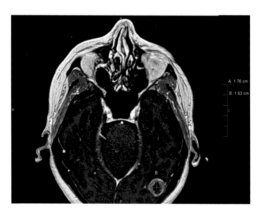

Answer

1. Based on Level 1 evidence, the options are SRS alone or surgery and WBRT. Based on ASTRO's 2014 Choosing Wisely statement, SRS alone is favored over SRS and WBRT in order to spare neurocognition. Another option is comfort measures only without brain radiation. His median survival based on the DS-GPA is 4.4 months.

Question

2. A 60-year-old patient with metastatic breast cancer, ER/PR negative Her2neu negative, presents with metastases to the brain, liver, and bone. Her KPS is 60. She has had numerous lines of chemotherapy and continues to have extra-cranial disease progression. A CT scan of brain shows multiple innumerable metastatic lesions throughout the brain. How would you treat this patient? What is her median overall survival?

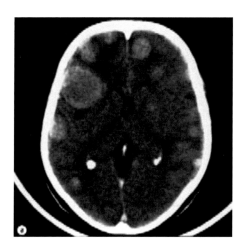

Answer

2. The patient may be considered for palliative WBRT (e.g., 2,000 cGy in 5-daily fractions or 3,000 cGy in 10-daily fractions). Another option is comfort measures only with the use of dexamethasone and no brain radiation therapy. Based on the DS-GPA, her median survival is 3.4 months.

Question

3. A 51-year-old man with BRAF positive metastatic melanoma presents with metastases to brain only. He presents with mild right sided weakness. He has two brain metastases (7.1-mm left frontal lobe and 8.3-mm left temporal lobe). His KPS is 90. What options are available to this patient? What is his median overall survival?

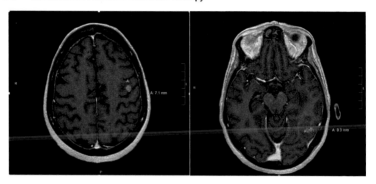

Answer

3. Radiosurgery alone is favored to treat the two small brain metastases. Based on the DS-GPA, his median survival is 8.8 months.

REFERENCES

1. Johnson JD, Young B. Demographics of brain metastasis. *Neurosurg Clin N Am*. 1996;7(3):337-344.
2. Barnholtz-Sloan JS, Sloan AE, Davis FG, et al. Incidence proportions of brain metastases in patients diagnosed (1973 to 2001) in the Metropolitan Detroit Cancer Surveillance System. *J Clin Oncol*. July 15, 2004;22(14):2865-2872.
3. Gaspar L, Scott C, Rotman M, et al. Recursive partitioning analysis (RPA) of prognostic factors in three Radiation Therapy Oncology Group (RTOG) brain metastases trials. *Int J Radiat Oncol Biol Phys*. 1997;37(4):745-751.
4. Sperduto PW, Chao ST, Sneed PK, et al. Diagnosis-specific prognostic factors, indexes, and treatment outcomes for patients with newly diagnosed brain metastases: a multi-institutional analysis of 4,259 patients. *Int J Radiat Oncol Biol Phys*. July 1, 2010;77(3):655-661.
5. Sperduto PW, Kased N, Roberge D, et al. Effect of tumor subtype on survival and the graded prognostic assessment for patients with breast cancer and brain metastases. *Int J Radiat Oncol Biol Phys*. April 1, 2012;82(5):2111-2117.
6. Ryken TC, McDermott M, Robinson PD, et al. The role of steroids in the management of brain metastases: a systematic review and evidence-based clinical practice guideline. *J Neurooncol*. January 2010;96(1):103-114.
7. Mulvenna PM, Nankivell MG, Barton R, et al. Whole brain radiotherapy for brain metastases from non-small cell lung cancer: quality of life (QOL) and overall survival (OS) results from the UK Medical Research Council QUARTZ randomised clinical trial (ISRCTN 3826061). *J Clin Oncol*. 2015;33(suppl 15):8005.
8. Langley RE, Stephens RJ, Nankivell M, et al. Interim data from the Medical Research Council QUARTZ Trial: does whole brain radiotherapy affect the

survival and quality of life of patients with brain metastases from non-small cell lung cancer? *Clin Oncol (R Coll Radiol)*. March 2013;25(3):e23-e30.

9. Horton J, Baxter DH, Olson KB. The management of metastases to the brain by irradiation and corticosteroids. *Am J Roentgenol Radium Ther Nucl Med*. 1971;111(2):334-336.

10. Kalkanis SN, Kondziolka D, Gaspar LE, et al. The role of surgical resection in the management of newly diagnosed brain metastases: a systematic review and evidence-based clinical practice guideline. *J Neurooncol*. January 2010;96(1):33-43.

11. Gaspar LE, Mehta MP, Patchell RA, et al. The role of whole brain radiation therapy in the management of newly diagnosed brain metastases: a systematic review and evidence-based clinical practice guideline. *J Neurooncol*. January 2010;96(1):17-32.

12. Patchell RA, Tibbs PA, Walsh JW, et al. A randomized trial of surgery in the treatment of single metastases to the brain. *N Engl J Med*. 1990;322:494-500.

13. Noordijk EM, Vecht CJ, Haaxma-Reiche H, et al. The choice of treatment of single brain metastasis should be based on extracranial tumor activity and age. *Int J Radiat Oncol Biol Phys*. 1994;29(4):711-717.

14. Mintz AH, Kestle J, Rathbone MP, et al. A randomized trial to assess the efficacy of surgery in addition to radiotherapy in patients with a single cerebral metastasis. *Cancer*. October 1, 1996;78(7):1470-1476.

15. Patchell RA, Tibbs PA, Regine WF, et al. Postoperative radiotherapy in the treatment of single metastases to the brain. *JAMA*. November 4, 1998;280(17).

16. Kocher M, Soffietti R, Abacioglu U, et al. Adjuvant whole-brain radiotherapy versus observation after radiosurgery or surgical resection of one to three cerebral metastases: results of the EORTC 22952-26001 study. *J Clin Oncol*. January 10, 2011;29(2):134-141.

17. Andrews DW, Scott CB, Sperduto PW, et al. Whole brain radiation therapy with or without stereotactic radiosurgery boost for patients with one to three brain metastases: phase III results of the RTOG 9508 randomised trial. *Lancet*. May 22, 2004;363(9422):1665-1672.

18. Aoyama H, Shirato H, Tago M, et al. Stereotactic radiosurgery plus whole-brain radiation therapy vs stereotactic radiosurgery alone for treatment of brain metastases. A randomized controlled trial. *JAMA*. 2006;295(21):2483-2491.

19. Chang EL, Wefel JS, Hess KR, et al. Neurocognition in patients with brain metastases treated with radiosurgery or radiosurgery plus whole-brain irradiation: a randomised controlled trial. *Lancet Oncol*. November 2009;10(11):1037-1044.

20. Hart MG, Grant R, Walker M, Dickinson H. Surgical resection and whole brain radiation therapy versus whole brain radiation therapy alone for single brain metastases (Review). *Cochrane Libr*. 2011;(3).

21. Brown PD, Asher AL, Karla VB, et al. NCCTG N0574 (Alliance): A phase III randomized trial of whole brain radiation therapy (WBRT) in addition to

radiosurgery (SRS) in patients with 1 to 3 brain metastases. *J Clin Oncol.* 2015;33(suppl 15):LBA4.

22. Yamamoto M, Serizawa T, Shuto T, et al. Stereotactic radiosurgery for patients with multiple brain metastases (JLGK0901): a multi-institutional prospective observational study. *Lancet Oncol.* March 7, 2014;2045(14):1-9.

23. Mehta MP. The controversy surrounding the use of whole-brain radiotherapy in brain metastases patients. *Neuro Oncol.* 2015;17(7):919-923.

24. Gondi V, Tomé WA, Mehta MP. Why avoid the hippocampus? A comprehensive review. *Radiother Oncol.* December 2010;97(3):370-376.

25. Brown PD, Pugh S, Laack NN, et al. Memantine for the prevention of cognitive dysfunction in patients receiving whole-brain radiotherapy: a randomized, double-blind, placebo-controlled trial. *Neuro Oncol.* 2013;15(10):1429-1437.

26. Rapp SR, Case LD, Peiffer A, et al. Donepezil for irradiated brain tumor survivors: a phase III randomized placebo-controlled clinical trial. *J Clin Oncol.* 2015;33(15):1653-1659.

27. Gondi V, Pugh SL, Tome WA, et al. Preservation of memory with conformal avoidance of the hippocampal neural stem-cell compartment during whole-brain radiotherapy for brain metastases (RTOG 0933): a phase II multi-institutional trial. *J Clin Oncol.* 2014;32(34):3810-3819.

28. Owonikoko TK, Arbiser J, Zelnak A, et al. Current approaches to the treatment of metastatic brain tumours. *Nat Rev Clin Oncol.* 2014;11(4):203-222.

29. Sperduto PW, Wang M, Robins HI, et al. A phase 3 trial of whole brain radiation therapy and stereotactic radiosurgery alone versus WBRT and SRS with temozolomide or erlotinib for non-small lung cancer and 1 to 3 brain metastases: Radiation Therapy Oncology Group 0320. *Int J Radiat Oncol Biol Phys.* 2013;85(5):1312-1318.

30. Ceresoli GL, Cappuzzo F, Gregorc V, et al. Gefitinib in patients with brain metastases from non-small cell lung cancer: a prospective trial. *Ann Oncol.* 2004;15(7):1042-1047.

31. Welsh JW, Komaki R, Amini A, et al. Phase II trial of erlotinib plus concurrent whole-brain radiation therapy for patients with brain metastases from non-small-cell lung cancer. *J Clin Oncol.* March 1, 2013;31(7):895-902.

32. Wu C, Li YL, Wang ZM, et al. Gefitinib as palliative therapy for lung adenocarcinoma metastatic to the brain. *Lung Cancer.* 2007;57(3):359-364.

33. Bachelot T, Romieu G, Campone M, et al. Lapatinib plus capecitabine in patients with previously untreated brain metastases from HER2-positive metastatic breast cancer (LANDSCAPE): a single-group phase 2 study. *Lancet Oncol.* January 2013;14(1):64-71.

34. Lin NU, Diéras V, Paul D, et al. Multicenter phase II study of lapatinib in patients with brain metastases from HER2-positive breast cancer. *Clin Cancer Res.* Feburary 15, 2009;15(4):1452-1459.

35. Long GV, Trefzer U, Davies MA, et al. Dabrafenib in patients with Val600Glu or Val600Lys BRAF-mutant melanoma metastatic to the brain

(BREAK-MB): a multicentre, open-label, phase 2 trial. *Lancet Oncol.* November 2012;13(11):1087-1095.

36. Dummer R, Goldinger SM, Turtschi CP, et al. Vemurafenib in patients with BRAFV600 mutation-positive melanoma with symptomatic brain metastases: final results of an open-label pilot study. *Eur J Cancer.* 2014;50(3):611-621.

37. Harding JJ, Catalanotti F, Munhoz RR, et al. A retrospective evaluation of vemurafenib as treatment for BRAF-mutant melanoma brain metastases. *Oncologist.* 2015;20(7):789-797.

38. Margolin K, Ernstoff MS, Hamid O, et al. Ipilimumab in patients with melanoma and brain metastases: an open-label, phase 2 trial. *Lancet Oncol.* May 2012;13(5):459-465.

39. Kiess AP, Wolchok JD, Barker CA, et al. Stereotactic radiosurgery for melanoma brain metastases in patients receiving ipilimumab: safety profile and efficacy of combined treatment. *Int J Radiat Oncol Biol Phys.* 2015;92(2):368-375.

40. Tsao MN, Lloyd N, Wong RK, et al. Whole brain radiotherapy for the treatment of newly diagnosed multiple brain metastases (Review). *Cochrane Libr.* 2012;(4).

41. Kohutek ZA, Yamada Y, Chan TA, et al. Long-term risk of radionecrosis and imaging changes after stereotactic radiosurgery for brain metastases. *J Neurooncol.* 2015;125(1):149-156.

42. Mikkelsen T, Paleologos NA, Robinson PD, et al. The role of prophylactic anticonvulsants in the management of brain metastases: a systematic review and evidence-based clinical practice guideline. *J Neurooncol.* 2010;96(1):97-102.

6   Head and Neck

Albert Tiong and June Corry

INTRODUCTION

Head and neck cancers encompass a wide variety of anatomic subsites and histologies, though most commonly they are squamous cell carcinomas arising from the oral cavity, pharynx, larynx, and skin. These tumors can cause significant distress for patients with symptoms including: pain, bleeding, obstructed breathing, cranial nerve palsies, and impaired speech and swallowing. Where cure is not possible, radiation therapy (RT) is an effective means to palliate many of these symptoms. Despite treatment, however, many patients will still die of their primary tumor, rather than from metastasis (unlike many other cancers). It is therefore imperative to control the locoregional disease and symptoms and also to ensure that patients do not spend the remaining part of their limited life spans recovering from treatment-related toxicities; for instance, a full course of radical RT to the head and neck region can take an average of 4 to 6 weeks to recover from acute toxicities.[1]

A head and neck cancer patient may be considered palliative because of the following reasons:

- Extent of disease where primary surgery and/or (chemo)RT is unlikely to cure the disease
- Poor performance status
- Comorbidities, which will preclude radical treatment and/or significantly reduce the life-expectancy of the patient
- Presence of distant metastatic disease

The decision to treat a patient with palliative versus curative intent can be difficult as both the disease and treatment-related toxicity produce significant symptoms. There is no simple, universally validated algorithm to predict the survival of these patients. Figure 6.1 provides an algorithm for decision making regarding radical versus palliative treatment. There are a number of prognostic factors that should be taken into account when making these decisions.

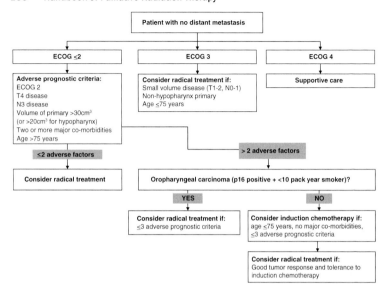

FIGURE 6.1 Algorithm for selecting patients with head and neck squamous cell carcinoma for radical treatment. ECOG, Eastern Cooperative Oncology Group.

Performance Status, Comorbidities, and Age

Performance status reflects the interaction between a patient's age, medical comorbidities, and tumor burden. While age is an adverse predictor of cause-specific survival, the effect appears to be modest.[2] Of greater importance is the presence of comorbidities, performance status of patients, and the impact of age on organ function and reserve, which have significant impact on the overall survival of patients.[3]

In patients who have become deconditioned as a result of tumors, several strategies may be employed in an attempt to improve their performance statuses. Improving a patient's nutritional status and pain medication regimen may facilitate curative treatment. Nutritional status can be addressed by appetite stimulants, enhancing protein intake, and addressing issues that interfere with oral intake. Placement of a nasogastric or percutaneous enterostomy feeding tube may be required. Induction chemotherapy may have the same effect by reducing the tumor burden. Although these strategies are yet to be validated in prospective trials, they are not uncommonly used in clinical practice.

Anatomic Subsite and Biological Markers

The potential curability of a tumor is highly influenced by the subsite of disease and presence of biological markers. For instance, undifferentiated nasopharyngeal carcinomas are known to be highly sensitive to both RT and chemotherapy and despite advanced locoregional disease, cure is still achievable.[4] Similarly, human papilloma virus (HPV) associated oropharyngeal carcinomas in nonsmokers can have high cure rates despite locally advanced disease.[5] Subsites such as the oral cavity and hypopharynx have traditionally been much more difficult to cure in very advanced disease; careful consideration of other prognostic signs should occur before considering radical treatment.

Stage and Volume of Disease

In general, the higher the stage of disease, the lower the locoregional control rates. The T- and N-stage, however, may not tell the whole story. The volume of disease is independently predictive of local control on multivariate analysis.[6] Patients with undifferentiated nasopharyngeal carcinomas and HPV-positive oropharyngeal carcinomas can have a high complete response rate to treatment despite high-volume disease.

Histology

Although squamous cell carcinoma is the most common histology in the head and neck, there are other rare entities that occur in this region. The selection of intensity of treatment is dictated by the natural time course of disease. For instance, adenoid cystic carcinomas have a high propensity to recur distantly but can have protracted courses with survival measured in years. It is therefore important not to undertreat the local disease sites and associated perineural areas of risk.[7]

Distant Metastasis

The presence of distant metastasis has traditionally meant that patients were considered incurable from their disease. This paradigm may be changing for selected patients. In patients with undifferentiated nasopharyngeal carcinoma and a limited number of distant metastasis, aggressive treatment can achieve very durable (more than 3 years) progression-free survival.[8–10] This may also apply to HPV-positive patients with distant metastasis.[11] In other subsites, there is currently not enough evidence to treat these patients aggressively.

Despite known prognostic factors, the decision to recommend radical treatment may be difficult. Performance status, stage, and volume of disease have the greatest impact on this treatment decision. Algorithms that incorporate clinical and disease factors to predict the survival of head and neck cancer patients after treatment are listed in Table 6.1. More general prognostic tools

TABLE 6.1 Some Published Algorithms for Predicting the Survival of Patients with Head and Neck Cancers

Subsite	Study	Comment
Oropharynx	Velazquez et al.[31] www.predictcancer.org	Prediction of 2- and 5-year survival of patients who were treated with 70 Gy/35 fractions of (chemo)RT based on Hb, gender, smoking, TN, p16 status, and comorbidities.
Oropharynx	Ang et al.[5]	Prediction of 3-year OS (low, intermediate, or high) of patients with oropharynx cancers based on p16 status, TN, and smoking pack-year. Only patients with good PS (Zubrod 0 or 1) were included in this study.
Oropharynx	Rietbergen et al.[32]	Prediction of 3-year OS (low, intermediate, or high) of patients with oropharynx cancer based on p16 status, TN, smoking pack-year, and ACE-27 comorbidity index.
Larynx	Egelmeer et al.[33] www.predictcancer.org	Nomogram to predict LC and OS of patients with glottic cancers who are treated with RT alone. Factors that were predictive were age, gender, TN, glottic versus non-glottic, Hb, and RT dose (in 2 Gy equivalent). Comorbidity data were not collected in this population and patients treated with chemotherapy were excluded.
Multiple mucosal subsites	Datema et al.[3]	Predictive model for survival based on inputs of age, gender, TNM, prior malignancy, ACE-27, and tumor subsite. Unfortunately, the interface is not freely available.
Multiple mucosal subsites	Wang et al.[34] http://skynet.ohsu.edu/ nomograms	Model for predicting OS if patient survives treatment from cancer at time points from completion of treatment. Data are based on SEER and hence crude (variables entered include race, site, sex, non-TNM stage, and grade).

ACE-27, adult comorbidity evaluation-27; Hb, hemoglobin; LC, local control; OS, overall survival; PS, performance status; RT, radiation therapy; SEER, Surveillance, Epidemiology, and End Results Program; TNM, tumor, nodal, and distant metastasis staging.

can be found in Chapter 2 and Appendix B. Ultimately, predicting whether a patient will tolerate radical treatment and achieve disease control depends on the clinical experience and acumen of the physician.

Multidisciplinary discussion that includes radiation oncologists, medical oncologists, surgeons, speech pathologists, dieticians, nurses, and social workers can facilitate treatment discussions. It is worthwhile to clarify the intent of treatment; whether it is for cure or palliation, how high or low the probability of cure, and whether the goal is to palliate current or imminent symptoms versus prolong disease control and possibly survival.

RT is an effective treatment for locoregional symptoms and produces a higher response rate when compared with chemotherapy.[12–26] Therefore, where local or regional disease is the predominant cause of patients' symptoms, RT should be used. Chemotherapy is the initial treatment approach when distant metastases predominate or if further radiation is limited because of prior treatment. Embarking on retreatment with RT in the head and neck should be made after careful consideration of the potential side effects versus the benefits. Median survival with full-dose irradiation (60 Gy) entails significant treatment-related morbidity (8%–10% grade 4 reactions) with somewhat limited survival (median survival 8–12 months).[28,29]

In the palliative setting, there are multiple trials using a wide range of different dose fractionation schedules. Table 6.2 summaries the current literature regarding RT in head and neck cancers. These trials show that RT is an effective means to palliate symptoms. As an example, palliative RT may achieve the following improvements:

- Pain (56%–67%)
- Dysphagia (33%–53%)
- Voice quality (31%–57%)

In the palliative context, the best RT regimen is an unanswered question. Unfortunately, trials in the palliative context are extremely heterogeneous with regard to clinical factors such as patient's age, performance status, and stage of disease. Hence, direct comparison of different regimens is difficult. What is clear, however, is that higher doses of radiation produce more side effects, with up to 65% grade 3 mucositis.[14] This may not be justified in a patient who will survive 6 to 9 months, as a considerable amount of time will be spent recovering from acute toxicities.

In those with very poor prognoses (i.e., <3 months survival), single fraction regimens (8 Gy), are preferred. If needed, the dose can be repeated twice more at weekly or so intervals. Single fractions are often used for

TABLE 6.2 Studies on palliative RT for HNSCC

Study	No. of Patients	RT regimen	Overall Survival	Objective Outcomes	Percentage of Patients with Subjective Outcome Improvements	Acute Toxicity
Prospective						
Fortin et al.[27]	32	25 Gy in 5 fractions over 1 week	Median 6.5 months	PFS 3.2 months	85% would have chosen to have RT again when asked	13% any grade 3 toxicity, 17% no toxicity at all
Ghoshal et al.[17]	15	14 Gy/4 fractions over 2 days, monthly × 3	Not specified	PR 67%, SD 13%, RR* 67%	Improved: pain 67%, dysphagia 33%	Grade 1 mucositis 40%, Grade 2 mucositis 13%, No grade 3 reactions
Agarwal et al.[16]	110	40 Gy/16 fractions over 3.5 weeks and further RT to 50 Gy if good response	Not specified	CR 10%, PR 63%, RR* 73% SD 16%	Improved: 74% of patients (individual symptoms not specified)	Grade 3 mucositis 63%, Grade 4 mucositis 3%, Grade 3 skin reaction 14%
Porceddu et al.[13]	35	30 Gy/5 fractions, 2 per week +/- 6 Gy boost	Median 6.1 months	CR 43%, PR 37%, RR* 80% SD 8.6%	Improved: pain 67%, dysphagia 33%, energy 29%	Grade 3 mucositis 26%, Grade 3 skin reaction 11%, Grade 3 dysphagia 11%
Corry et al.[12]	30	14 Gy/4 fractions over 2 days, monthly × 3	Median 5.7 months	CR 7%, PR 47%, RR* 54% SD 23%	Improved: pain 56%, dysphagia 33%, hoarseness 31%	Grade 2 mucositis 11%, Grade 2 xerostomia 37%, No Grade 3 toxicities
Mohanti et al.[15]	505	20 Gy/5 fractions over 1 week (352 patients) and further RT up to biological equivalent of 70 Gy in responders (153 patients)	Median 6.7 months for lower dose and 13.3 months for high dose	CR 10%, PR 37%, RR* 47% SD not specified	Improved: pain 57%, dysphagia 53%, hoarseness 57%	Grade 3 skin reaction 56%, Grade 3 mucositis 62%, (in higher dose group)

TABLE 6.2 Studies on Palliative RT for HNSCC (*continued*)

Study	No. of Patients	RT regimen	Overall Survival	Objective Outcomes	Percentage of Patients with Subjective Outcome Improvements	Acute Toxicity
Paris et al.[18]	37	14.8 Gy/4 fractions over 2 days, every 3 weeks × 3	Average 4.5 months	CR 28%, PR 49%	Improved: 85% of patients (individual symptoms not specified)	Toxicity not graded
Retrospective						
Beek et al.[26]	81	48 Gy in 12 fractions (3–4 fractions per week)	Median 7.2 months	CR/MR/PR 72%	"Positive palliative effect" 63%	Grade 3–5 mucositis in 70%
Kancherla et al.[21]	33	40 Gy/10 fractions over 4 weeks with a 2 week mid-treatment break	Median 9 months	CR 39%, PR 33%, RR* 72%	Improved: 79% of patients (individual symptoms not specified)	Grade 3 skin reaction 3%, Grade 3 mucositis 6%, Grade 3 esophageal toxicity 9%
Stevens et al.[19]	148	Multiple regimens (50 Gy/20 fractions, 24 Gy/3 fractions, 60 Gy/25 fractions, 30 Gy/10 fractions, 60 Gy/30 fractions, 70 Gy/35 fractions)	Median 5.2 months	A RR* 82%, MR 6%, NR or PD 12%	Improved: 85% of patients (individual symptoms not specified and information on only 65% of patients)	Not collected

(*continued*)

TABLE 6.2 Studies on Palliative RT for HNSCC (*continued*)

Study	No. of Patients	RT Regimen	Overall Survival	Objective Outcomes	Percentage of Patients with Subjective Outcome Improvements	Acute Toxicity
Al-Mamgani et al.[14]	158	50 Gy/16 fractions, 5 per week	Median 17 months	CR 45%, PR 25%, RR* 70% SD 6%	Improved: pain 77%, dysphagia 65% (information in only 40% of patients)	Grade 3 mucositis 65%, Grade 3 skin reaction 45%, Grade 3 dysphagia 45%
Chen et al.[20]	311	Multiple regimens (14 Gy/4 fractions × 3, 70 Gy/35 fractions, 30 Gy/10 fractions, 37.5 Gy/15 fractions, 20 Gy/5 fractions)	Survival 3 to 8 months depending on regimen	Not specified	60% to 86% of patients had a "palliative response" (no standardized measure)	≥ Grade 3 reaction varied from 9% with 14 Gy/4 fractions to 38% for 70 Gy/35 fractions
Erkal et al.[22]**	40	30 Gy/10 fractions daily or 20 Gy/2 fractions weekly	Not specified	CR 12%, PR 76%, RR* 86	Complete response in symptoms 18%, partial response in symptoms 76%	Not specified

CR, complete response; HNSCC, head and neck squamous cell carcinoma; MR, mixed response; PD, progressive disease; PFS, progression-free survival; PR, partial response; RR, response rate (CR + PR); RT, radiation therapy; SD, stable disease.

*RR = CR + PR

**Only included patients with squamous cell carcinoma involving cervical lymph nodes with unknown primary

Source: Adapted with permission from Lutz S, Chow E, Hoskin PJ. *Radiation Oncology in Palliative Cancer Care.* John Wiley & Sons; 2013.

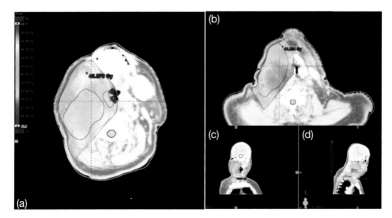

FIGURE 6.2 Simple conformal technique to deliver palliative radiation therapy (RT; QUAD shot) for a T1N3 SCC right tonsil in an 82-year-old male with multiple comorbidities, ECOG 3. (a) Tonsil level, (b) lower neck level, (c) coronal view, (d) sagittal view.

bleeding or pain but are unlikely to produce durable local control. For patients with a predicted survival of 3 to 9 months we recommend the QUAD shot (14 Gy in 4 fractions, twice per day over 2 days or daily over 4 consecutive days, and repeated monthly for a total of three times) or a similar hypofractionated regimen. This regimen demonstrated effective palliation of symptoms with minimal toxicity (10% grade 2 mucositis and no grade 3 toxicity; Figure 6.2).[12] For patients with a predicted survival of more than 9 months, higher doses (EQ2 for late toxicity of 55 Gy equivalent or more) may be justified as trials suggest a better tumor response (e.g., 45% complete response rate with 50 Gy in 16 fractions compared with no complete responses in the QUAD shot study). The addition of concurrent chemotherapy in the palliative context has been explored but it is uncertain whether this provides additional benefit.[30]

TREATMENT PLANNING

Immobilization

Patients are positioned supine with a thermoplastic mask fixed at five points in most instances. This is to ensure that treatment is reproducible and that planning target volume (PTV) margins can be kept minimal (5–10 mm) to minimize acute toxicities.

CT scanning

Patients are CT scanned with a standard image acquisition (3 mm slices). For lower dose treatments (e.g., QUAD shot) we do not use contrast. In most instances the tumor can be seen well enough on diagnostic imaging and slightly larger margins may be used to account for delineation uncertainties. Where higher doses are used, IV contrast can be justified to assist in delineation. Where resources are limited, two-dimensional simulation with field border markings is used instead.

Target Volume Delineation

Gross tumor (primary and nodes likely to be symptomatic in the lifetime of the patient) should be delineated. When available, imaging modalities acquired in the work-up of the patient should be used (either side by side or with fusion).

Prophylactic nodal irradiation (PNI) in general is not warranted. It may be considered in situations where high-dose palliation is used, where there is a reasonable chance of complete or near complete response in the gross disease. In this setting, an untreated node may progress and become symptomatic, and reirradiation might be difficult. We recommend that treatment volumes cover a single echelon of lymph nodes on either side of the gross disease. PNI needs to be considered in the context of potential toxicity. Where the potential side effects are low (e.g., lower neck field), then it may be justified. If toxicity is likely to be increased significantly (e.g., treating bilaterally through midline structures), then the benefit of PNI should be weighed against the additional morbidity. Irradiating gross disease will produce the most clinical benefit.

In general, the PTV should be a 5 to 10 mm expansion on the gross tumor volume (GTV). Whether a clinical target volume (CTV) should be used in the palliative context to cover potential microscopic spread is debatable. Figure 6.2 shows an example of a typical volume and dosimetric coverage for a QUAD shot.

Normal Organ Tolerances

Given the limited life spans of patients with metastatic head and neck cancer, late effects are unlikely to cause problems. However, with palliative regimens, dose constraints are used for organs at risk where late effects could have potentially devastating consequences. For example, with the QUAD shot regimen, we limit the maximum point dose to the spinal cord to 28 Gy, which is easily achievable in most instances. Where the tumor lies close to critical structures, the underdosing of the GTV needs to be weighed against the clinical likelihood of late toxicity. Late toxicity with most palliative regimens is unlikely to occur in patients with life expectancies of less than 6 months. Other normal structures to be mindful of include the oral cavity and midline structures (larynx, pharynx) and major salivary glands. The dose to these structures should be minimized to reduce acute toxicity, which can affect quality of life.

Dose Solutions

In resource-limited environments, the simplest field arrangement should be used (e.g., parallel opposed or three-field plans). This also has the advantage of limiting the time for which the patient has to be on the treatment couch. Where resources are available, intensity-modulated radiation therapy (IMRT) has the potential to spare some toxicity.[26] In our experience, a QUAD shot in most instances produces minimal mucositis with conformal treatment and IMRT would not add a significant benefit. If higher doses are prescribed, IMRT is much more likely to add a clinical benefit by sparing organs such as the parotid glands and midline structures.

Dose-Fractionation

Based on published literature and institutional experience we suggest the following as a guide (though there are many other dose-fractionation schedules that are acceptable):

- Prognosis less than 3 months: best supportive care or short courses that may help with bleeding or pain (8 Gy, which may be repeated at day 7 and day 21, total dose 24 Gy).
- Prognosis 3 to 9 months: 14 Gy in 4 fractions; two fractions per day over 2 days (at least 6 hours apart) or daily over 4 consecutive days. This may be repeated two times on a monthly basis. This treatment can improve a patient's current symptoms or delay/prevent symptoms that may happen in the future.
- Prognosis more than 9 months: 50 Gy in 20 fractions to palliative symptoms and potentially prolong survival.

TOXICITY

Acute side effects to RT in the head and neck region include:

- Radiation dermatitis
  - Xerostomia
- Dysgeusia
- Painful mucositis
- Edema—With large tumors within the oral cavity, pharynx, or larynx, there is the potential for edema and obstruction from hypofractionated regimens. Prophylactic steroids may be used as a precaution.

Serious late toxicities are only likely to be problematic for patients living more than 6 months. Late toxicities could potentially include:

- Xerostomia
- Skin fibrosis
- More significant long-term side effects such as osteonecrosis of the mandible, dysphagia, and feeding tube dependency are more likely to be seen in high-dose regimens (EQ2 for late reaction tissues of more than 55 Gy)
- Spinal cord toxicity is a very uncommon issue in this population of patients with limited life spans

SYMPTOM MANAGEMENT

Although RT is effective at reducing the symptoms associated with tumor, the following are useful adjuncts for symptoms (either from cancer or treatment):

- Analgesia: topical analgesia (e.g., lignocaine viscous) is useful for oral and pharyngeal pain to provide short-term relief (e.g., just prior to food), or systemic agents, such as acetaminophen, non-steroidal anti-inflammatory drugs, and opioids.
- Bleeding: absorbent and pressure dressings, tranexamic acid
- Obstructed breathing: steroids are useful for providing short-term relief (e.g., dexamethasone 8 mg daily). Tracheostomies should rarely be used. Though a tracheostomy may minimally increase survival, quality of life is diminished due to local effects of tumors and the potential for fungation of tumors through tracheostomy tubes. This is an important medical scenario that needs proactive medical discussion in relevant patients.
- Dysphagia: the prolongation of life as a result of assisted feeding may be outweighed by the resultant poor quality of life. Steroids may again be used to improve swallowing temporarily by reducing tumor-related edema. Patients and their caregivers need to be actively involved in this discussion as they are easier to insert than remove.
- Timing is of the essence, but patients need opportunities to discuss and document their wishes regarding end-of-life care plans.
- Facilitation of access to local palliative care services (e.g., nursing, medical equipment for the home)

CASES WITH SELF-ASSESSMENT AND QUESTIONS

Case 6.1: Metastatic Disease

Question

A 70-year-old man has stable metastatic prostate carcinoma (diagnosed 2 years ago with three involved sites—sacrum, L3, and ilium; Figure 6.3) and T3N0 larynx cancer (Figure 6.4a and b). Of the following, which would be the most appropriate treatment?

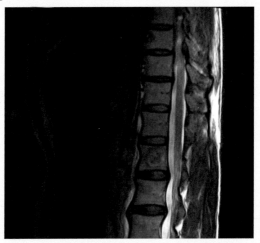

FIGURE 6.3 Magnetic resonance image of the sclerotic focus of prostate cancer at L3.

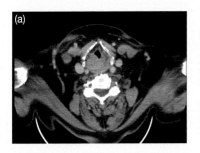
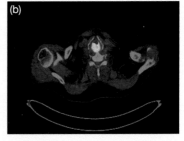

FIGURE 6.4 Computed tomography (a) and PET-CT (b) axial image at the level of the larynx.

1. Total laryngectomy
2. Laser debulking
3. Radical (chemo)RT (e.g., 70 Gy in 35 fractions)
4. Palliative radiotherapy (e.g., QUAD shot)
5. Palliative chemotherapy

Answer

3. There are some circumstances, even in the setting of metastatic disease, where aggressive treatment is warranted. A patient with stable metastatic prostate carcinoma is likely to have a prognosis measured in years. Untreated T3 larynx cancer is likely to progress in less than 3 months. Palliative RT or chemotherapy would likely provide a progression-free survival of 5 to 6 months. It is therefore important to consider treating the larynx cancer aggressively to ensure that it does not cause significant symptoms and limit his life expectancy. With combination (chemo)RT in appropriately selected patients, 80% to 90% of patients will achieve a complete response with voice preservation. The period of toxicity is likely to be short (3 months) compared with his prognosis from metastatic prostate carcinoma (measured in years).

Case 6.2: Poor Performance Status Patient

Question

A 50-year-old woman with multiple comorbidities including an acquired brain injury from alcohol abuse presented with a T4a hypopharynx SCC with odynophagia and a weight of 40 kg. She is capable of only borderline self-care, and has limited social support and an ECOG performance status of 2 (Figure 6.5a and b).

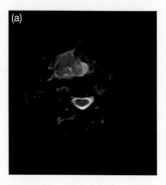 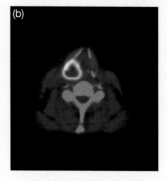

FIGURE 6.5 Axial MR (a) and PET-CT (b) images at the level of the hypopharynx.

What would be the most appropriate treatment?

1. Total pharyngo-laryngectomy
2. Laser debulking
3. Radical (chemo)RT
4. Palliative chemotherapy
5. Palliative RT (e.g., QUAD shot)

Answer

5. It is often difficult to decide between radical or palliative treatment for patients. However, a patient who is unable to manage a tracheostomy after pharyngo-laryngectomy or self-manage the acute toxicities from (chemo)RT poses a high treatment mortality risk. The curability of locally advanced disease in a poor prognostic site is not high, even in a fit patient. While often a difficult decision to make in a relatively young patient, the best treatment will be palliative to provide symptom relief without significant toxicity in her likely short life span.

Case 6.3: Volume of Treatment

Question

An 85-year-old man presents with an 8 cm left neck node (level 2–4; Figure 6.6a and b), which is causing some pain and discomfort. Work-up including a thorough skin examination, nasoendoscopic examination, and CT neck and chest do not reveal a primary, contralateral neck nodes, or distant metastatic disease. He is a heavy ex-smoker, has chronic obstructive pulmonary disease (COPD) with an exercise tolerance of 30 m, and his performance status is ECOG 3. He is unsuitable for general anesthesia. You have opted for a hypofractionated palliative RT regimen. What would be an appropriate CTV to cover his disease?

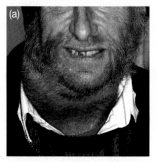 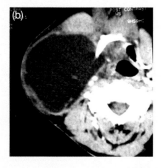

FIGURE 6.6 (a) Photograph of the large right neck mass; (b) CT axial image of the neck mass.

1. CTV should include the gross nodal disease, putative primary sites including nasopharynx, oropharynx, hypopharynx, and larynx, and contralateral neck
2. CTV should include gross nodal disease and a reduced volume of putative primary sites (oropharynx and hypopharynx) and contralateral neck
3. CTV should include gross nodal disease and contralateral neck only
4. CTV should include only gross nodal disease

Answer

4. While this patient is likely to have an occult primary in his pharyngeal axis, given the radiological and endoscopic findings, there is a low chance of a symptomatic primary emerging in his limited lifetime. A hypofractionated palliative RT regimen will reduce his pain and discomfort but is unlikely to produce a complete tumor response with an 8 cm tumor. Therefore, treating large volumes of the pharyngeal axis will lead to added toxicity with very little therapeutic gain.

CLINICAL PEARLS

- Many patients with head and neck cancer will die of their primary tumors rather than from metastasis. It is therefore imperative to control the locoregional disease and symptoms, and also to ensure that patients do not spend the remaining parts of their limited life spans recovering from treatment-related toxicities.
- Despite known prognostic factors, the decision to recommend radical treatment may be difficult. Performance status, stage, and volume of disease have the greatest impact on this treatment decision (Figure 6.1). Algorithms that incorporate clinical and disease factors to predict the survival of head and neck cancer patients after treatment are listed in Table 6.1.
- For patients with a predicted survival of 3 to 9 months, we recommend the QUAD shot (14 Gy in 4 fractions, twice per day over 2 days or daily over 4 consecutive days, and repeated monthly for a total of three times) or a similar hypofractionated regimen. This regimen palliates symptoms with minimal toxicity.
- Gross tumor (primary and nodes likely to be symptomatic in the lifetime of the patient) should be delineated and encompassed in treatment fields.

REFERENCES

1. Mehanna H, West C, Nutting C, Paleri V. Head and neck cancer—Part 2: Treatment and prognostic factors. *BMJ*. 2010;341:c4690.
2. Huang SH, O'Sullivan B, Waldron J, et al. Patterns of care in elderly head-and-neck cancer radiation oncology patients: a single-center cohort study. *Int J Radiat Oncol Biol Phys*. 2011;79(1):46-51.
3. Datema FR, Ferrier MB, van der Schroeff MP, de Jong B, Robert J. Impact of comorbidity on short-term mortality and overall survival of head and neck cancer patients. *Head Neck*. 2010;32(6):728-736.
4. Lee AW, Yau T, Wong DH, et al. Treatment of stage IV (A-B) nasopharyngeal carcinoma by induction-concurrent chemoradiotherapy and accelerated fractionation. *Int J Radiat Oncol Biol Phys*. 2005;63(5):1331-1338.
5. Ang KK, Harris J, Wheeler R, et al. Human papillomavirus and survival of patients with oropharyngeal cancer. *N Engl J Med*. 2010;363(1):24-35.
6. Knegjens JL, Hauptmann M, Pameijer FA, et al. Tumor volume as prognostic factor in chemoradiation for advanced head and neck cancer. *Head Neck*. 2011;33(3):375-382.
7. Fordice J, Kershaw C, El-Naggar A, Goepfert H. Adenoid cystic carcinoma of the head and neck: predictors of morbidity and mortality. *Arch Otolaryngol Head Neck Surg*. 1999;125(2):149-152.
8. Hui EP, Leung SF, Au JS, et al. Lung metastasis alone in nasopharyngeal carcinoma: a relatively favorable prognostic group. *Cancer*. 2004;101(2):300-306.
9. Fandi A, Bachouchi M, Azli N, et al. Long-term disease-free survivors in metastatic undifferentiated carcinoma of nasopharyngeal type. *J Clin Oncol*. 2000;18(6):1324-1330.
10. Cheng L, Sham J, Chiu C, et al. Surgical resection of pulmonary metastases from nasopharyngeal carcinoma. *Aust N Z J Surg*. 1996;66(2):71-73.
11. Huang SH, Perez-Ordonez B, Weinreb I, et al. Natural course of distant metastases following radiotherapy or chemoradiotherapy in HPV-related oropharyngeal cancer. *Oral Oncol*. 2013;49(1):79-85.
12. Corry J, Peters LJ, D'Costa I, et al. The "QUAD SHOT"—a phase II study of palliative radiotherapy for incurable head and neck cancer. *Radiother Oncol*. 2005;77(2):137-142.
13. Porceddu SV, Rosser B, Burmeister BH, et al. Hypofractionated radiotherapy for the palliation of advanced head and neck cancer in patients unsuitable for curative treatment—"Hypo Trial". *Radiother Oncol*. 2007; 85(3):456-462.
14. Al-Mamgani A, Tans L, Van Rooij PH, et al. Hypofractionated radiotherapy denoted as the "Christie scheme": an effective means of palliating patients with head and neck cancers not suitable for curative treatment. *Acta Oncol*. 2009;48(4):562-570.
15. Mohanti BK, Umapathy H, Bahadur S, et al. Short course palliative radiotherapy of 20 Gy in 5 fractions for advanced and incurable head and neck cancer: AIIMS study. *Radiother Oncol*. 2004;71(3):275-280.

16. Agarwal JP, Nemade B, Murthy V, et al. Hypofractionated, palliative radiotherapy for advanced head and neck cancer. *Radiother Oncol.* 2008;89(1):51-56.

17. Ghoshal S, Chakraborty S, Moudgil N, et al. Quad shot: a short but effective schedule for palliative radiation for head and neck carcinoma. *Indian J Palliat Care.* 2009;15(2):137-140.

18. Paris KJ, Spanos WJ, Lindberg RD, et al. Phase I–II study of multiple daily fractions for palliation of advanced head and neck malignancies. *Int J Radiat Oncol Biol Phys.* 1993;25(4):657-660.

19. Stevens CM, Huang SH, Fung S, et al. Retrospective study of palliative radiotherapy in newly diagnosed head and neck carcinoma. *Int J Radiat Oncol Biol Phys.* 2011;81(4):958-963.

20. Chen AM, Vaughan A, Narayan S, Vijayakumar S. Palliative radiation therapy for head and neck cancer: toward an optimal fractionation scheme. *Head Neck.* 2008;30(12):1586-1591.

21. Kancherla K, Oksuz D, Prestwich R, et al. The role of split-course hypofractionated palliative radiotherapy in head and neck cancer. *Clin Oncol (R Coll Radiol).* 2011;23(2):141-148.

22. Erkal HS, Mendenhall WM, Amdur RJ, et al. Squamous cell carcinomas metastatic to cervical lymph nodes from an unknown head and neck mucosal site treated with radiation therapy with palliative intent. *Radiother Oncol.* 2001;59(3):319-321.

23. Vermorken JB, Mesia R, Rivera F, et al. Platinum-based chemotherapy plus cetuximab in head and neck cancer. *N Engl J Med.* 2008;359(11):1116-1127.

24. Forastiere AA, Shank D, Neuberg D, et al. Final report of a phase II evaluation of paclitaxel in patients with advanced squamous cell carcinoma of the head and neck: an Eastern Cooperative Oncology Group trial (PA390). *Cancer.* 1998;82(11):2270-2274.

25. Samlowski WE, Moon J, Kuebler JP, et al. Evaluation of the combination of docetaxel/carboplatin in patients with metastatic or recurrent squamous cell carcinoma of the head and neck (SCCHN): a Southwest Oncology Group Phase II study. *Cancer Invest.* 2007;25(3):182-188.

26. Beek KM, Kaanders JH, Janssens GO, et al. Effectiveness and toxicity of hypofractionated high-dose intensity-modulated radiotherapy versus 2-and 3-dimensional radiotherapy in incurable head and neck cancer. *Head Neck.* April 2015;38(suppl 1): E1264-E1270.

27. Fortin B, Khaouam N, Filion E, et al. Palliative radiation therapy for advanced head and neck carcinomas: a phase 2 study. *Int J Radiat Oncol Biol Phys.* 2016;95(2):647-653.

28. Spencer SA, Harris J, Wheeler RH, et al. Final report of RTOG 9610, a multi-institutional trial of reirradiation and chemotherapy for unresectable recurrent squamous cell carcinoma of the head and neck. *Head Neck.* 2008;30(3):281-288.

29. Langer CJ, Harris J, Horwitz EM, et al. Phase II study of low-dose paclitaxel and cisplatin in combination with split-course concomitant twice-daily

reirradiation in recurrent squamous cell carcinoma of the head and neck: results of Radiation Therapy Oncology Group Protocol 9911. *J Clin Oncol.* 2007;25(30):4800-4805.

30. Minatel E, Gigante M, Franchin G, et al. Combined radiotherapy and bleomycin in patients with inoperable head and neck cancer with unfavourable prognostic factors and severe symptoms. *Oral Oncol.* 1998;34(2):119-122.

31. Velazquez ER, Hoebers F, Aerts HJ, et al. Externally validated HPV-based prognostic nomogram for oropharyngeal carcinoma patients yields more accurate predictions than TNM staging. *Radiother Oncol.* 2014;113(3):324-330.

32. Rietbergen MM, Brakenhoff RH, Bloemena E, et al. Human papillomavirus detection and comorbidity: critical issues in selection of patients with oropharyngeal cancer for treatment de-escalation trials. *Ann Oncol.* 2013;24(11):2740-2745.

33. Egelmeer AG, Velazquez ER, de Jong JM, et al. Development and validation of a nomogram for prediction of survival and local control in laryngeal carcinoma patients treated with radiotherapy alone: a cohort study based on 994 patients. *Radiother Oncol.* 2011;100(1):108-115.

34. Wang SJ, Wissel AR, Ord CB, et al. Individualized estimation of conditional survival for patients with head and neck cancer. *Otolaryngol Head Neck Surg.* 2011;145(1):71-73.

7 Lung and Central Airway Malignancies

Sarah Baker and Alysa Fairchild

INTRODUCTION

Lung cancer remains the leading cause of cancer mortality worldwide, with 1.8 million patients diagnosed in 2012.[1] 75% to 85% of patients with lung cancer present with disease too advanced to be treated with curative intent.[2] The majority of patients with advanced lung cancer have symptoms amenable to palliation with radiation therapy (RT)[3]; for example, 20% to 30% will develop airway obstruction at some point during their disease course.[4] Additionally, lung metastases develop in 20% to 54% of extrathoracic malignancies, commonly from breast and colorectal primaries, and may also become symptomatic enough to require RT.[5]

Palliative thoracic RT is therefore a key component of the care of many patients. RT can be indicated in the clinical scenarios of airway obstruction, hemoptysis, cough, chest pain, dyspnea, hoarseness, Horner's syndrome, and superior vena cava obstruction (SVCO), contributing to improvements in quality of life (QoL). This chapter summarizes the literature surrounding dose and fractionation, techniques, toxicities, and outcomes of palliative thoracic RT delivered for these common indications, as well as briefly describes essential supportive care considerations. Although the majority of the available literature describes non–small-cell lung cancer (NSCLC), many aspects of the following chapter, such as pretreatment optimization and technical factors, are applicable to the palliative treatment of small cell lung cancer (SCLC) and lung metastases. Consolidative thoracic RT after systemic therapy in extensive stage SCLC will also be discussed.

WHICH PATIENTS WITH STAGE IV NSCLC CAN BE TREATED AGGRESSIVELY?

While patients with metastatic disease are nearly always only candidates for palliative-intent treatment, there is a small proportion of patients with stage IV NSCLC—approximately 7%[6]—who either present with oligometastases or are rendered oligometastatic after palliative systemic therapy. While the specific definition of oligometastases varies, it is often taken as fewer than five discrete lesions outside of the primary site.[7] High-dose local RT (typically delivered as stereotactic body radiation therapy [SBRT]) results in high treated metastasis control rates, delaying progression, and allowing continued systemic treatment. However, the topic of SBRT for oligometastases is beyond the scope of this chapter as the goal of RT in that situation is long-term disease control rather than palliation of symptoms. Excellent review articles on SBRT of lung metastases are available.[8–10]

WHICH PATIENTS WITH STAGE III NSCLC CANNOT BE TREATED AGGRESSIVELY?

The most robust prognostic factors in NSCLC are stage of disease, involuntary weight loss over the previous 3 to 6 months, and performance status (PS).[10] In general, patients with Eastern Cooperative Oncology Group (ECOG) PS greater than 2, weight loss greater than 10% over the last 3 months, or tumor size greater than 8 cm[11,12] are not likely to tolerate radical treatment—either surgery or definitive RT.[13] In patients with stage III disease with poor prognostic factors who cannot be treated for cure, a recent phase III trial investigated combined modality therapy, which incorporated hypofractionated RT. A total of 191 patients were randomized to concurrent chemoradiotherapy (42 Gy in 15 fractions starting with cycle two of chemotherapy) versus carboplatin and vinorelbine alone. The combined modality arm had significantly improved median overall survival (12.6 vs. 9.7 months) and long term QoL, but experienced more frequent hospital admissions (49% vs. 25%; $P < .01$) for treatment-related side effects including esophagitis and infection.[14]

EMERGENCY RADIATION THERAPY FOR SVCO AND AIRWAY COMPROMISE

SVCO from direct invasion or extrinsic compression is attributable to lung cancer 50 to 70% of the time.[15–18] Ten percent of all patients with SCLC, and 2% to 4% of those with NSCLC, will develop SVCO at some point in their disease trajectories.[15–18] Thrombosis as a contributor to SVCO syndrome is becoming more common due to the increased prevalence of intravascular devices such as catheters and pacemakers,[15,19] and it often coexists with malignancy-associated obstruction due to vascular hold-up. If thrombus is present, anticoagulation should be initiated,[20] but there is no evidence supporting its prophylactic use in the absence of other indications. Additional considerations include the placement of an endovenous stent, usually by interventional radiology, followed by RT; it is unclear at present whether long-term anticoagulation is also required.[21]

For more proximal mainstem or tracheal obstruction, especially in the context of stridor, rapid debulking can be provided through bronchoscopic ablation or laser, where resources exist, followed by urgent RT.[22–24] Occasionally, stenting, intubation, or tracheostomy may be required. Intraluminal stents provide symptom relief approximately 90% of the time.[23,25–27]

In cases of severe respiratory symptoms including stridor, patients require stabilization before RT to decrease the risk of acute decompensation on the treatment couch, and to mitigate symptoms in the interval before expected onset of benefit from RT, which ranges anywhere from 72 hours to a more typical 1 to 2 weeks.[22] RT-induced edema can transiently exacerbate symptoms. While there is no level 1 evidence supporting steroid use for airway obstruction or SVCO, steroids may temporize the transient worsening of symptoms due to treatment, preventing a serious situation from becoming disastrous.

WHAT FIRST: PALLIATIVE RADIATION THERAPY OR PALLIATIVE SYSTEMIC THERAPY?

Both in general and in the setting of SVCO specifically, the addition of concurrent chemotherapy has not been conclusively shown to improve response rates, locoregional control, symptomatic relief, or survival.[28–31] Therefore, palliative RT and palliative systemic therapy are almost always given sequentially, with advantages and disadvantages to each approach (Table 7.1).

Assuming no indication exists for emergency thoracic RT, patients ineligible for curative-intent treatment should be reviewed in a multidisciplinary rounds setting, so a consensus recommendation on an appropriate sequence of therapy can be reached (Table 7.2). This is essential, especially with a nonsquamous NSCLC patient with a tumor that is epidermal growth factor receptor- or anaplastic lymphoma kinase-mutated, which carry additional options for therapeutic intervention. The importance of obtaining a tissue biopsy prior to initiation of therapy cannot be overstated.

WHO SHOULD NOT BE TREATED WITH PALLIATIVE THORACIC RADIATION THERAPY?

Patients with an estimated life expectancy less than 1 month are not expected to derive substantial symptom improvement from thoracic RT, which often takes 4 to 6 weeks for full benefits to manifest. The time, inconvenience, and potential acute side effects of RT are not offset by significant improvements in symptomatology in that situation, and best supportive care should be the approach of choice. The exception is hemoptysis, which will often respond or resolve within a few days.[37]

TABLE 7.1 Advantages and Disadvantages of RT and Systemic Therapy as Initial Palliative Treatment Modalities

Modality	Advantages	Disadvantages	References
RT	▪ Addresses established or impending SVCO or airway obstruction urgently ▪ In moderate airway obstruction, may improve aeration to decrease the likelihood of infectious pneumonia during systemic therapy ▪ May be the only option in patients who are not candidates for systemic therapy due to age, PS, comorbidities, uncontrolled brain metastases, or absence of driver mutations ▪ Improvement of symptoms and PS from RT may allow some patients to become candidates for systemic therapy	▪ Widely disseminated disease outside the irradiated field is likely to progress during RT ▪ Delay to initiation of systemic therapy imposed by RT-associated toxicity ▪ Still controversial as to whether thoracic RT carries a survival benefit ▪ Thoracic RT in incurable but asymptomatic patients does not prevent future development of symptoms	Rowell and Gleeson,[22] Sundstrom et al.,[32] and Falk et al.[33]
Systemic therapy	▪ Simultaneously addresses all sites of extracranial disease ▪ Survival benefits in stage IV NSCLC and extensive stage SCLC for responders ▪ Does not carry the same risk of pulmonary side effects, which may be a consideration for a patient with poor baseline lung function/oxygen dependence ▪ Excellent response rates to targeted agents for those with driver mutations ▪ Responses may delay the need for RT	▪ More widespread and potentially more severe side effects ▪ More stringent eligibility criteria	Pfister et al.,[34] Davidoff et al.,[35] and Slotman et al.[36]

NSCLC, non–small-cell lung cancer; PS, performance status; RT, radiation therapy; SCLC, small cell lung cancer; SVCO, superior vena cava obstruction.

TABLE 7.2 Patient Selection for Palliative Thoracic RT: Factors to Consider

General	■ Patients should be reviewed at multidisciplinary tumor board and considered for systemic therapy as well as RT. ■ Informed consent must be obtained.
Patient factors	■ Confirmatory histology should be obtained prior to treatment whenever possible. ■ Evaluate prognostic factors such as weight loss and PS in order to estimate life expectancy. ■ Assess patient factors which may impact on treatment planning such as degree of orthopnea.
Disease factors	■ Patients should have symptomatic locoregional disease or radiologic evidence of an impending catastrophic event such as SVCO or tracheobronchial obstruction. ■ Rule out nonmalignant causes of symptoms. ■ Address reversible etiologies of symptoms prior to initiating RT if possible, by instituting supportive measures concurrently, including referral to specialists or allied health professionals. ■ Baseline symptom severity should not be so great that acute RT toxicities could be life threatening.

PS, performance status; RT, radiation therapy; SVCO, superior vena cava obstruction.

Thoracic RT in asymptomatic but incurable NSCLC provides no survival benefit and does not definitively prevent future development of symptoms, and may in fact reduce short term QoL due to acute side effects.[32,33] The risks and benefits of short course RT should be discussed with the patient, as proceeding is likely worthwhile only in the situation of impending airway, neurological, or vascular compromise (Table 7.3).

Patients with confusion (delirium or dementia) may not be able to tolerate coming to the cancer center for multiple daily visits. Short fractionation regimens and simple setup positions should be employed with additional immobilization measures as required. Assessment of ability to give informed consent is essential.

Although no specific criteria exist for minimum pre-RT pulmonary function, patients with poor lung function have less resilience for lung toxicity, and any complications that do occur may be more serious and potentially life-threatening. Baseline pulmonary function testing should be performed if the patient can tolerate them, and RT should be delivered with caution if the FEV1 and/or diffusing capacity of the lung for carbon monoxide (DLCO) are less than 20% of predicted values for age and gender. The need for supplemental oxygen is not a contraindication for palliative lung RT, especially when required for a reversible etiology such as a pulmonary embolus or pneumonia.

TABLE 7.3 Advantages and Disadvantages of Different Palliative RT Schedules

	Examples (Dose/fractions)	Advantages	Disadvantages	Consider in
Short course	16–17 Gy/2 1 week apart; 10 Gy/1	■ More convenient for patients and caregivers ■ More cost-effective ■ Less resource-intensive ■ Possibility of more rapid symptom palliation	■ Potential for higher incidence of myelopathy ■ Slightly increased rate of retreatment	■ Poor PS ■ Patients who live at a distance geographically
Longer course	30–35 Gy/10; 40–42 Gy/15; 45–50 Gy/20	■ Less reirradiation ■ Possible increase in 1 year OS by 4.8% if BED ≥35 Gy	■ Less convenient ■ Increased acute and subacute toxicity	■ Good PS ■ Willing to risk greater toxicity

BED, biologically equivalent dose; OS, overall survival PS, performance status; RT, radiation therapy.

However, degree of both dyspnea and orthopnea should be evaluated at the time of the initial physical examination to ensure these symptoms will not compromise a patient's ability to lie supine and still. Arrangements for continuous oxygen during set-up and treatment will help increase patient comfort.

It should be noted that patients should not be deemed poor RT candidates on the basis of advanced age alone. Surveillance, Epidemiology, and End Results Medicare linked data suggests an age-related disparity in the receipt of palliative RT in the United States, even after controlling for confounding covariates such as PS.[38] However, when controlling for stage and PS, age is not an independent predictor of worse outcome, nor are older patients less likely to complete a prescribed course of palliative thoracic RT.[39]

PRERADIATION THERAPY OPTIMIZATION

Several steps may be taken to optimize a patient's status prior to initiation of therapy, to increase their comfort as well as the likelihood of completing the RT, such as short course steroids or supplemental oxygen (Table 7.2). Consider thoracentesis for pleural effusion, and treating acute concurrent illness such as postobstructive or aspiration pneumonia. Abdominal distension can reduce lung volumes and contribute to dyspnea and can be alleviated by treating constipation or performing paracentesis for ascites. Medical optimization of active comorbid illnesses such as congestive heart failure (CHF) or chronic obstructive pulmonary disease (COPD) via appropriate specialist referral may be helpful, especially if it can be performed without undue delay. For patients with pain, a short-acting opioid can ease transfer on and off the simulation and treatment couch, and help ensure that patients are comfortable enough to remain still during treatment. Opioids are also useful to address breathlessness and cough. Anxiolytics could be considered for anxiety or claustrophobia associated with an immobilization shell.

Case 7.1: Radiation Therapy in the Setting of Ventilation

A 75-year-old woman with biopsy-confirmed stage IV NSCLC presents to her radiation oncology consultation in respiratory distress. She is agitated, using accessory muscles of respiration with three to four word dyspnea despite 4 L of oxygen. She has not been able to take in solid food for a number of weeks due to significant dysphagia, requiring emergency department visits for intravenous hydration, most recently 48 hours prior. She has lost 40 lb. in the last 3 months. On enhanced CT scan of the chest, there is an 8 cm mediastinal mass invading the esophagus and compressing both mainstem bronchi. She is stage IV on the basis of contralateral pulmonary nodules consistent with metastatic lesions and ECOG PS is 3 to 4.

What are the appropriate initial steps with this patient?

- Ensure that the patient is stable by performing vital signs in the clinic.
- Admit for symptom control including oxygen titration, opioids, nutritional bypass (feeding tube placement, if appropriate), and initiation of steroids. Consider a proton pump inhibitor or H2 blocker for gastric protection as well as inhaled bronchodilators. Proceeding with RT immediately could exacerbate her respiratory distress due to radiation-induced swelling.
- Palliative care consultation should be undertaken.

Despite the aforementioned interventions, over the next 2 days, the patient's breathing worsens and her oxygen saturation falls to 81% to 84% on 15 L.

What is the optimal management?

- Transfer to an acute care setting for stenting of the left mainstem bronchus. After the procedure, she remained intubated and ventilated in the Intensive Care Unit.

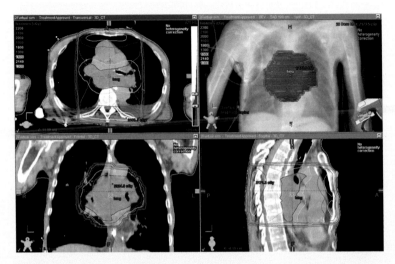

FIGURE 7.1 Case 1 contours and dose distribution. After insertion of a left mainstem bronchus stent, the patient received the first four fractions of emergency thoracic RT while intubated. Red: GTV. Cyan: PTV. Beam arrangement: parallel opposed. Energy: 6MV. Beam modifiers: multilieaf collimation. Dose fractionation schedule: 30 Gy/10 on consecutive days including the weekend.

If the patient is stable, can she proceed to RT?

■ Palliative RT can be initiated while intubated, and this patient completed 4 of 10 planned fractions in this manner, transported on a daily basis between hospitals (Figure 7.1). After extubation, she completed the prescribed 30 Gy in 10 fraction course without difficulty.

■ By the 2 month follow-up visit, she was no longer on supplemental oxygen, denied dyspnea or dysphagia, and was regaining weight. She went on to receive four cycles of cytotoxic systemic therapy with an excellent clinical and radiographic response.

OUTCOMES AFTER PALLIATIVE THORACIC RADIATION THERAPY

The dose required for optimal symptom palliation and whether higher doses improve survival or provide more durable local control are issues that have been addressed in several randomized controlled trials (RCTs). Table 7.4 summarizes the results of a recent meta-analyses.

In general, thoracic RT provides effective symptom palliation for hemoptysis, cough, and chest pain (Table 7.5). Dyspnea can be more refractory to

TABLE 7.4 Meta-analyses of Dose Fractionation Schedules for Palliative Thoracic RT

Meta-Analysis References	Patients Dose Schedules (Dose/fractions)	Comparison	Results
Stevens et al.[*,40]	N = 3,576 10 Gy/1–60 Gy/30	More versus fewer fraction regimens	∎ No difference in 1 year OS, symptom palliation, QoL, radiological response assessed by chest x-ray, esophagitis, or pneumonitis ∎ Relative risk of myelopathy with more fractions: 1.29 (95% CI 0.37 to 4.51)
Fairchild et al.[41]	N = 3,473 10 Gy/1–60 Gy/30	Regimens delivering ≥35 Gy_{10} BED versus <35 Gy_{10} BED	∎ Regimens ≥35 Gy_{10} BED associated with: • Significantly higher rate of improved total symptom score (77% vs. 65%, P = .003) • No difference in palliation of hemoptysis, cough, chest pain • 4.8% increase in 1 year OS (P = .002) • Increase in physician-assessed dysphagia (20.5% vs. 14.9%, P = .01) • Nonsignificant reduction in rate of thoracic reirradiation

BED, biologically equivalent dose; OS, overall survival; QoL, quality of life; RT, radiation therapy.

[*]Update of Cochrane meta-analyses originally published in 2001 and 2006.

RT as it is often multifactorial; in fact, up to 25% of dyspenic cancer patients lack obvious lung involvement.[45] Atelectasis secondary to airway obstruction and symptoms related to neurological compromise such as hoarseness may not normalize following RT, particularly if present for an extended duration prior to treatment.

TABLE 7.5 Symptom Response After Palliative Thoracic RT. Refers to NSCLC Unless Stated Otherwise

Symptom	Complete Response	Any Improvement	Number Needed to Treat	References
Hemoptysis	69%–74%	80%–81%	1.25	Fairchild et al.[41] and Samant and Gooi[42]
Chest pain	52%–58%	64%–65%	1.43	Fairchild et al.[41] and Samant and Gooi[42]
Cough	28%–32%	48%–54%	NR	Fairchild et al.[41]
SVCO	NR	60% NSCLC 77%–80% SCLC	1.3	Hohloch et al.[17], Rowell and Gleeson[22], and Samant and Gooi[42]
Dyspnea	NR	41%–66%	NR	MRC Lung Cancer Working Party[43,44]

MRC, Medical Research Council; NR, not reported; NSCLC, non–small-cell lung cancer; RT, radiation therapy; SCLC, small cell lung cancer; SVCO, superior vena cava obstruction.

The onset of symptom improvement varies from several days in the case of hemoptysis to approximately 2 to 4 weeks for most other symptoms.[22,46,47] RT-induced edema can exacerbate cough and dyspnea for the first 1 to 2 weeks following treatment, particularly with more hypofractionated schedules such as 17 Gy/2 fractions one week apart or 10 Gy/1 fraction.[46,47] While one or two fraction regimens may be associated with acute esophagitis, they may also contribute to more rapid onset of palliation.[46,47] A retrospective review of SVCO due to any histology reported that 3 Gy or more per fraction resulted in higher rates of symptom relief at 2 weeks than conventional fractionation.[29]

The duration of symptom improvement is a difficult endpoint to ascertain with certainty due to varying follow-up schedules, heterogeneous (or absent) symptom assessment, and poor patient survival overall. Reports describe improvements in total symptom score lasting approximately 22 weeks following RT,[46] to lasting at least 50% of the patient's remaining survival.[43,44,48]

There is no strong evidence that higher dose schedules result in longer lasting control of symptoms.[40]

Case 7.2: Radiation Therapy for Superior Vena Cava Obstruction

A 71-year-old woman with a sustained complete response to treatment 5 years prior for a stage IV follicular non-Hodgkin lymphoma presents with bilateral arm and neck swelling, headache, cough, and dyspnea. She is not in respiratory distress. Enhanced CT of the chest and upper abdomen demonstrates an 11 cm heterogeneous right upper lobe mass causing almost complete obstruction of the SVC. There is dilation of the azygous venous system with extensive superficial collateral veins apparent. Transthoracic needle core biopsy confirms poorly differentiated adenocarcinoma.

What treatment should she receive?

- She is stable and does not require emergency stent placement or airway stabilization.
- She was treated with 20 Gy/5 fractions (Figure 7.2) and experienced complete resolution of her symptoms 6 days after completing RT.

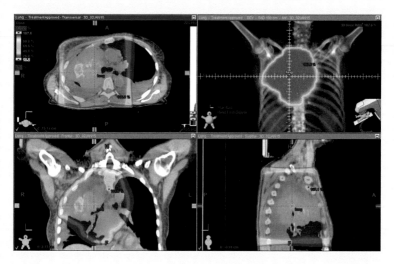

FIGURE 7.2 Example of treatment planning for SVCO. Beam arrangement: parallel opposed. Energy: 15 MV. Beam modifiers: multileaf collimation. Dose fractionation schedule: 20 Gy/5 fractions on consecutive days including the weekend. Weekend treatment may not be necessary at these fraction sizes.

TREATMENT PLANNING

Positioning, Immobilization, and Simulation

Set-up reproducibility will be improved via taking measures to maximize patient comfort (see the aforementioned pre-RT optimization). Conventional fluoroscopic two-dimensional (2D) simulation can be utilized in an after-hours emergency,[13] although the 3D data provided by CT simulation will decrease the likelihood of geographic miss and should be used whenever possible (Table 7.6). Patients are generally positioned supine with arms above the head to preserve the option of using oblique or lateral fields (to prevent unnecessary dose to the arms). Some will not be able elevate their arms due to restricted range of motion of the shoulders or poor respiratory function, and treating with the arms down is acceptable. In those patients with orthopnea that precludes lying flat, treatment on an incline on a breast board or using a positioning wedge, custom polyurethane foam, or evacuated vacuum cushions can be explored in consultation with simulation and dosimetry staff. Several institutions have developed devoted treatment chairs for this purpose.[49]

Target Delineation

In most palliative plans, the target volume is the symptomatic tumor rather than all gross and potential subclinical disease (Table 7.6). While treating additional macroscopic and microscopic disease may be considered in an effort to prevent future symptoms, as a rough estimation, these "elective" volumes should be included only if the treated volume can be limited to less than 200 cm^2.[13] Shielding should be liberally applied to critical structures to decrease the likelihood of acute side effects, which may compromise QoL in the short term.

Target and Normal Tissue Doses

Commonly used regimens include 30 Gy/10 fractions, 20 Gy/5 fractions, as well as 17 Gy/2 fractions 1 week apart and 10 Gy/1 fraction. In general, no particular schedule provides better symptom palliation or survival compared to others, as individual trials are conflicting; therefore, shorter courses are preferred for their advantages for the patient, caregiver, and department resources. Although it is unlikely that one course of palliative RT will exceed the tolerance doses of normal structures, commonly accepted normal tissue constraints presume standard fractionation.[50,51] When determining the tolerability and acceptability of a palliative thoracic RT plan, especially in the reirradiation setting, fraction size must be taken into account.

TABLE 7.6 Treatment Planning Recommendations for Palliative Thoracic RT

Simulation	■ Perform CT simulation with appropriate immobilization, such as a wing board ■ Intravenous contrast is rarely required
Gross tumor volume	■ Encompass the tumor which is causing symptoms, not necessarily all gross disease, since smaller volumes will decrease potential acute toxicity ■ Consider including disease that may cause symptoms in the future depending on volume of normal tissue in the field
Clinical target volume	■ Not required ■ May add 0.5–1 cm margin to GTV ■ Consider including ipsilateral central airways, mediastinum, and hilum
Planning target volume	■ Institution-specific but often 0.5–1 cm margin on CTV (or 1–2 cm margin on GTV) ■ Consider larger margin in cranio-caudal direction due to respiratory motion if not addressed otherwise
Dose	■ Consider hypofractionation to decrease overall treatment time, depending on estimated risk of toxicity ■ Limit spinal cord, lung volume receiving 20 Gy or more, and mean lung doses
Beam arrangement and energy	■ Simple field arrangements are preferred as they are faster to plan and faster to deliver ■ Ensure adequate shielding of spinal cord especially in large dose per fraction courses (≥3 Gy) ■ Photon beams in the range of 4–15 MV are generally used
Dose and position verification	■ Consider employing port films, electronic portal verification, and/or in vivo dosimetry as necessary, especially in a reirradiation or high-dose palliation setting

CTV, clinical target volume; GTV, gross tumor volume; RT, radiation therapy.

Energy

Lower energy photon beams have traditionally been preferred due to a sharper penumbra and more rapid dose build up in the low-density lung.[52] Higher energy beams, however, are able to obtain deeper penetration and better dose uniformity. Utilization of a dose-calculation algorithm that accurately accounts for heterogeneities allows for the construction of plans with either low or high energy without a clinically significant difference in plan quality.[53]

Beam Arrangement

Basic beam arrangements such as an anteroposterior posteroanterior (APPA) parallel opposed pair (POP) are most frequently used in the palliative setting and allow for more efficient planning, reduced use of departmental resources, and more rapid treatment delivery than more complicated planning techniques. A POP plan through the mediastinum also minimizes entrance and exit doses to lung parenchyma. The dosimetric advantages provided by more complex beam arrangements and intensity-modulated RT (IMRT) are not likely to be relevant in the palliative setting except in very specific circumstances such as

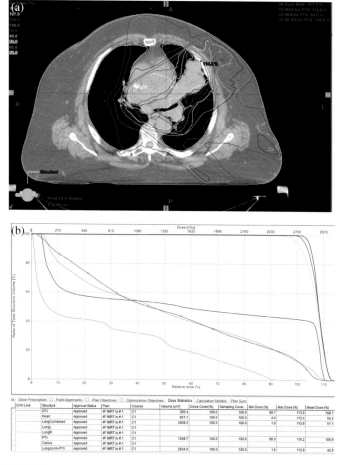

FIGURE 7.3 (a) Dose distribution from an IMRT palliative thoracic RT plan. (b) Dose-volume histogram. Red: GTV. Cyan: PTV.

reirradiation (ReRT), treating a high-dose target near a critical structure, or a large tumor in the setting of small lung volumes[37,54] (Figure 7.3).

EXTENSIVE STAGE SCLC POSTCHEMOTHERAPY

A recent phase 3 RCT demonstrated improved outcomes with the addition of consolidative thoracic RT (30 Gy/10 fractions), following any response to four to six cycles of standard cytotoxic chemotherapy, in extensive-stage SCLC (Figure 7.4). All patients received prophylactic cranial irradiation. Compared to patients who did not receive thoracic RT, those treated with radiation had

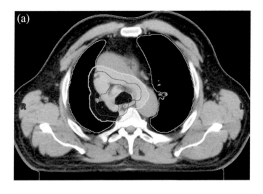

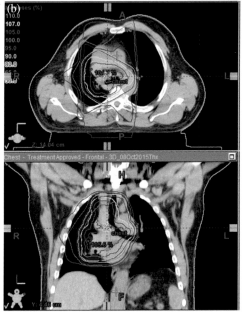

FIGURE 7.4
Consolidative RT volumes (a) and dose distribution (b) after chemotherapy response in extensive stage small cell lung cancer. Note that this is an example of a situation where a CTV is employed since the target includes the prechemotherapy extent of hilar and mediastinal adenopathy, along with the postchemotherapy residual disease elsewhere. Red: GTV. Purple: CTV. Cyan: PTV. Beam arrangement: 3DCRT (4 field). Energy: 15MV. Beam modifiers: wedges. Dose fractionation schedule: 30 Gy/10.

significant increases in 2-year overall survival (13 % vs. 3%) and 6-month progression-free survival (24% vs. 7%). Thoracic RT was well-tolerated, with a nonsignificant increase in grade 3 fatigue only (4.5% vs. 3.2%).[36]

REIRRADIATION

The need for thoracic reirradiation (ReRT) is common, particularly in patients with lung cancer, due to high rates of local failure even after curative-intent therapy.[54] Traditionally, concerns over high rates of toxicity from cumulative RT dose led to a reluctance to utilize ReRT. Recent publications, however, suggest that with careful dose calculation and planning, including generating a composite plan to calculate additive dose to critical structures, ReRT can be safe and effective at symptom palliation.[55–57] Rates of toxicity may be higher and efficacy lower than initial thoracic RT, and patients should be advised of such.[55,57] A long interval between initial RT and ReRT may be a good predictor for a better outcome, suggesting a more indolent cancer and also a lower risk of cumulative toxicity. A minimum of 3 months from initial RT is recommended. Patients whose disease progressed during initial RT are not likely to benefit from ReRT.[57]

A recent literature review of 13 publications on thoracic ReRT for lung cancer reported a range of doses from 12 to 70 Gy (median 36 Gy) and a 69% rate of symptom improvement. Reported esophagitis and pneumonitis rates were 17% and 12% respectively, with RT complications contributing to 2% of deaths.[57] An earlier review reported high rates of symptom palliation with short courses of 20 to 30 Gy.[58] A retrospective review of 78 NSCLC patients reirradiated with 8 Gy/1 fraction demonstrated an 86% response rate for chest pain lasting for a median duration of 6.1 months, with an approximate 5% risk of grade 3 pneumonitis.[55]

The main indication for endobronchial brachytherapy (EBB) is for patients previously treated with external beam RT who have symptomatic endobronchial recurrence or progression causing dyspnea or cough.[59–62] EBB involves bronchoscopic placement of a radioactive source (usually Iridium-192) in close proximity to an endobronchial tumor. Two Cochrane meta-analyses have not demonstrated benefit from either EBB alone for palliation of symptoms, or from the addition of EBB to external beam RT.[61,63]

Case 7.1 Revisited

The patient is rereferred by her medical oncologist after progressing through first-line cytotoxic chemotherapy (four cycles of carboplatin/vinorelbine) and 2 months of second-line erlotinib. It has been 18 months since her first course of RT (30 Gy/10 fractions). She has redeveloped chest pain and cough. CT scan has confirmed progression in the form of a 4.4 cm subcarinal lesion and new bilateral pleural effusions.

Is it reasonable to offer further mediastinal RT?

ReRT carries with it a greater risk of acute, subacute, and late side effects than the first course of RT. It is uncertain how potentially radioresponsive her in-field progression is, given the exposure to both previous RT and systemic therapy. However, in the absence of other options, ReRT could be offered with the goals of improving chest pain and cough. After discussing the potential risks and benefits, she decides to proceed with ReRT (Figure 7.5). She was prescribed 16 Gy/8 fractions delivered via a POP beam arrangement with shielding to decrease the dose to the esophagus, spinal cord, and surrounding lung. A composite plan was generated and showed a V20 of 26.6%, maximum cord dose of 43.3 Gy, and mean esophagus dose of 36 Gy.

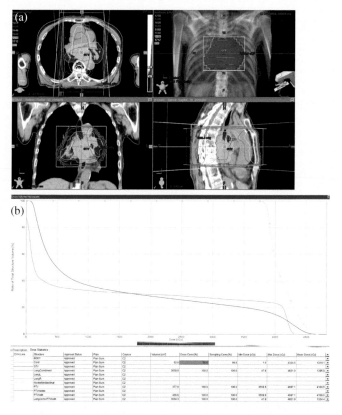

FIGURE 7.5 Case 1 revisited. Plan sum shows both courses of thoracic RT. (a) Composite dose distribution. (b) Composite DVH. Second course beam arrangement: parallel opposed. Energy: 6 MV. Beam modifiers: multilieaf collimation. Dose fractionation schedule: 16 Gy/8.

What are some potential late toxicities?

▪ One month following RT, she had experienced a complete response in terms of resolution of central chest pain and cough. However, she had developed dysphagia. A swallowing study suggested a mid-esophageal stricture. She was referred to gastroenterology for dilatation.

RADIATION THERAPY TOXICITY AND SYMPTOM MANAGEMENT

Symptoms of RT-induced toxicity can be similar to the symptoms of recurrent disease or comorbid illness, and these should be ruled out before presuming they are RT side effects.[64] Patients should be evaluated at least weekly during palliative thoracic RT for acute toxicity and supportive medication titration. The first follow-up appointment should be approximately 6 weeks after completion of RT for early assessment of symptom status and to screen for RT pneumonitis. Follow-up thereafter may be performed by the treating radiation oncologist, medical oncologist, or primary care physician.

Palliative thoracic RT is generally well-tolerated. Factors which increase the risk of RT toxicity include the volume of tissue irradiated, total dose, fraction size, concurrent systemic therapy, and comorbidities such as COPD. Acute toxicities are common but generally self-limited or resolvable with medical management and supportive care. Late toxicities are rare after palliative RT, but are often difficult to treat or irreversible.

Acute toxicities typically begin during the course of treatment and resolve within 1 to 2 weeks of RT completion (Table 7.7). Radiation-induced fatigue is common and poorly understood. Exacerbating factors including anemia, sleep disturbance (e.g., secondary to steroids), chemotherapy, and psychological stressors should be addressed.[67] Skin toxicity is limited to the RT field and usually consists of mild erythema, pruritus, or dry skin.[69] Dysphagia secondary to esophagitis is the most frequent in-field side effect of palliative thoracic RT[40,41] and can lead to complications such as malnutrition, dehydration, and aspiration if severe.[69] Subclinical pericarditis or pericardial effusion may occur, and are often found incidentally on follow-up radiological investigations.[64] Pneumonitis can present with dyspnea, cough, and low-grade fever, typically 6 to 12 weeks following RT (Figure 7.6), although it is still relatively uncommon in relation to infectious or aspiration pneumonia.

Late effects (generally taken to mean 3 or more months after completion of RT) are uncommon due to the limited life expectancy of many patients as well as the lower total dose of most palliative regimens.[42] L'hermitte's sign (paresthesia with neck flexion) is transient and typically occurs within 6 months of RT which has encompassed parts of the cervical or thoracic

TABLE 7.7 Acute and Subacute Side Effects of Palliative Thoracic RT

Toxicity	Incidence	Management Suggestions	References
Acute			
Fatigue	Common	▪ Supervised exercise program ▪ Modification of exacerbating factors ▪ No specific pharmacologic intervention is evidence based	Rorth et al.[65]
Esophagitis	Mild 34% Moderate-severe 10%	▪ Dietary modifications ▪ Oral rinses–sodium bicarbonate ▪ Antifungals–mycostatin ▪ Analgesics in elixir form, viscous xylocaine, "Pink Lady," benzydamine mouthwash ▪ Sucralfate suspension ▪ Treatment of associated acid reflux ▪ Fluid supplementation and electrolyte correction	Fairchild et al.,[41] Spiro et al.,[64] and Metcalfe et al.[66]
Nausea	Not common unless left lower lobe treated	▪ Antiemetics ▪ H2 blockers	Howell[70]
Subacute			
Pneumonitis	2%–4%*	▪ Prednisone 60–100 mg/day × 2 weeks	Fairchild et al.[41] and Spiro et al.[64]

RT, radiation therapy.
*Reported incidence depends on RT dose.

spinal cord. Esophageal submucosal fibrosis can result in stricture, ulceration, or perforation.[64,70] Pulmonary fibrosis evolves over 6 to 24 months and may contribute to dyspnea, cough, decreased exercise tolerance, and requirement for supplemental oxygen. Treatment is supportive with no

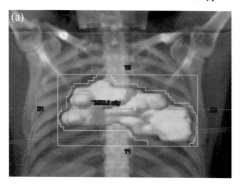

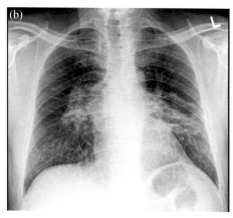

FIGURE 7.6
Radiation pneumonitis after 30 Gy/10 palliative thoracic RT. (a) Depiction of PTV and field borders. (b) Chest x-ray 11 weeks later demonstrating consolidation corresponding to the field borders.

intervention of proven benefit.[64] Myelopathy is a serious potential toxicity secondary to demyelination, necrosis, and vasculopathy, and can result in paraplegia.[64] Estimated rates are generally less than 0.5%[40,41]; it is unclear at present whether there is a correlation with RT dose. When reirradiating or treating with palliative RT after a curative dose, particular attention should be paid to spinal cord dose and off-cord techniques should be strongly considered.

SUMMARY

Palliative thoracic RT can provide effective symptom palliation and improve QoL for patients with incurable malignancies. While shorter RT regimens may be more convenient for patients and caregivers, longer regimens may provide a modest survival advantage in patients with good PS with a potential trade-off of increased likelihood of side effects. The caveat to this is that none of these studies were powered to detect differences in survival. Optimizing a patient's status prior to RT with supportive measures and treating underlying comorbidities can increase the likelihood of a patient successfully completing RT.

SELF-ASSESSMENT

Questions

1. What would you consider the minimum life expectancy to offer a patient with palliative thoracic RT?
   A. ≥1 month
   B. ≥3 months
   C. ≥6 months
   D. ≥12 months
   E. No minimum life expectancy

2. How would you rate the effectiveness of RT for the treatment of the following cancer-related symptoms? *(Please check most appropriate response.)*

	Not Effective	Somewhat Effective	Very Effective	Don't Know
Airway obstruction				
Hemoptysis				
Superior vena cava obstruction				
Dysphagia				
Upper limb edema from axillary surgery				

3. True/False: Longer courses of radiation are associated with longer survival in the treatment of metastatic lung cancer.

4. Which of the following generally precludes radical treatment in stage III lung cancer?
   A. Age greater than 70
   B. Tumor stage T3
   C. Karnofsky performance score (KPS) 50 (ECOG 3)
   D. Unintentional weight loss

1. A. Life expectancy should be ≥1 month for palliative thoracic RT since radiation takes time for the palliative effects to be realized. The exception is hemoptysis, for which a response within 24 to 48 hours can be seen. For hemoptysis, there is no minimum life expectancy.

2. Individual patient responses vary. For airway obstruction, superior vena caval obstruction and dysphagia palliative radiation is somewhat to very effective depending on the series. Palliative radiation is very effective at relieving hemoptysis and not effective at relieving edema caused by surgery.

	Not Effective	Somewhat Effective	Very Effective	Don't Know
Airway obstruction		✓	✓	
Hemoptysis			✓	
Superior vena cava obstruction		✓	✓	
Dysphagia		✓	✓	
Upper limb edema from axillary surgery	✓			

3. False: None of the studies that have looked at fractionation in lung cancer were powered to detect differences in survival. There have been several studies that demonstrate longer survival with longer fractionation but others that found the opposite. In addition, some of the trials included patients with stage III disease that were not clearly metastatic but had tumors that were thought too large, or patients who were too frail for curative treatment, as well as those with poor prognostic features. For patients who were medically frail or with stage III disease too advanced for cure, longer courses of palliative radiation may be more appropriate.

4. C. Patients with KPS less than 50 or ECOG greater than 2 are unlikely to be able to tolerate concurrent chemoradiation with curative intent. Age itself is not a poor prognostic factor. Weight loss greater than 10% of body weight in the last 3 months is a poor prognostic factor. T3 tumors, if larger than 8 cm, may preclude tolerance of radical treatment but T3 tumors can be T3 by virtue of invasion into the chest wall, mediastinal pleura, or diaphragm, proximity to the carina, multiple nodules in the same lobe, or size larger than 7 cm.

CLINICAL PEARLS

- The most robust prognostic factors in NSCLC are stage of disease, involuntary weight loss over the previous 3 to 6 months, and PS. In general, patients with ECOG PS greater than 2, weight loss greater than 10% over the last 3 months, or tumor size larger than 8 cm are not likely to tolerate radical treatment—either surgery or definitive RT.
- Patients with an estimated life expectancy less than 1 month are not expected to derive substantial symptom improvement from thoracic RT, which often takes 4 to 6 weeks for its full benefits to manifest. The time, inconvenience, and potential acute side effects of RT are not offset by significant improvements in symptomatology in that situation, and best supportive care should be the approach of choice. The exception is hemoptysis, which will often respond or resolve within a few days.
- Thoracic RT provides effective symptom palliation for hemoptysis, cough, dyspnea, and chest pain. Dyspnea can be more refractory to RT as it is often multifactorial.
- Commonly used dose fractionation regimens include 30 Gy/10, 20 Gy/5, 17 Gy/2 1 week apart, and 10 Gy/1. In general, no particular schedule provides better symptom palliation or survival compared to others, as individual trials are conflicting; therefore, shorter courses are preferred for their advantages for the patient, caregiver, and department resources.

REFERENCES

1. Brambilla E, Travis WD. Lung cancer. In: Stewart BW, Wild CP, eds. *World Cancer Report*. Lyon: World Health Organization; 2014.
2. National Lung Cancer Audit Project Team. National Lung Cancer Audit 2013. Health and Social Care Information Centre December 2013.
3. Chute CG, Greenberg ER, Baron J, et al. Presenting conditions of 1539 population-based lung cancer patients by cell type and stage in New Hampshire and Vermont. *Cancer*. 1985;56(8):2107-2111.
4. Theodore PR. Emergent management of malignancy-related acute airway obstruction. *Emerg Med Clin North Am*. 2009;27(2):231-241.
5. Mohammed TL, Chowdhry A, Reddy GP, et al. ACR appropriateness criteria® screening for pulmonary metastases. *J Thorac Imaging*. 2011;26(1):W1-3.
6. Pfannschmidt J, Dienemann H. Surgical treatment of oligometastatic non-small cell lung cancer. *Lung Cancer*. 2010;69(3):251-258.

7. Badakhshi H, Grun A, Stromberger C, et al. Oligometastases: the new paradigm and options for radiotherapy. A critical review. *Strahlenther Onkol.* 2013;189(5):357-363.

8. Tree A, Khoo VS, Eeles RA, et al. Stereotactic body radiotherapy for oligometastases. *Lancet Oncol.* 2013;14(1):E28-37.

9. Lo S, Moffatt-Bruce SD, Dawson LA, et al. The role of local therapy in the management of lung and liver oligometastases. *Nat Rev Clin Oncol.* 2011;8(7):405-416.

10. Timmerman R, Bizekis CS, Pass HI, et al. Local surgical, ablative, and radiation treatment of metastases. *CA Cancer J Clin.* 2009;59(3):145-170.

11. Brundage MD, Davies D, Mackillop WJ. Prognostic factors in non-small cell lung cancer. *Chest.* 2002;122(3):1037-1057.

12. Bradley JF, Ieumwananonthachai N, Purdy JA, et al. Gross tumor volume, critical prognostic factor in patients treated with three-dimensional conformal radiation therapy for non-small-cell lung carcinoma. *Int J Radiat Oncol Biol Phys.* 2002;52(1):49-57.

13. Dehing-Oberije C, de Ruysscher D, van der Weide H, et al. Tumor volume combined with number of positive lymph node stations is a more important prognostic factor than TNM stage for survival of non-small-cell lung cancer patients treated with (chemo) radiotherapy. *Int J Radiat Oncol Biol Phys.* 2008;70(4):1039-1044.

14. Sundstrom S. Palliative external beam thoracic radiation therapy of non-small cell lung cancer. In: Jeremic B, ed. *Advances in Radiation Oncology in Lung Cancer.* Heidelberg: Springer, 2011.

15. Strøm HH, Bremnes RM, Sundstrøm SH, et al. Concurrent palliative chemo-radiation leads to survival and quality of life benefits in poor prognosis stage III non-small-cell lung cancer: a randomised trial by the Norwegian Lung Cancer Study Group. Br J Cancer. 2013;109(6):1467-1475.

16. Rice TW, Rodriguez RM, Light RW. The superior vena cava syndrome: clinical characteristics and evolving etiology. *Medicine (Baltimore).* 2006;85(1):37-42.

17. Wan JF, Bezjak A. Superior vena cava syndrome. *Emerg Med Clin North Am.* 2009;27(2):243-255.

18. Hohloch K, Bertram N, Trumper L, et al. Superior vena cava syndrome caused by a malignant tumor: a retrospective single-center analysis of 124 cases. *J Cancer Res Clin Oncol.* 2014;140(12):2129-2134.

19. Chan RC, Chan YC, Cheng SW. Mid- and long-term follow-up experience in patients with malignant superior vena cava obstruction. *Interact Cardiovasc Thorac Surg.* 2013;16(4):455-458.

20. Chee CE, Bjarnason H, Prasad A. Superior vena cava syndrome: an increasingly frequent complication of cardiac procedures. *Nat Clin Pract Cardiovasc Med.* 2007;4(4):226-230.

21. Debourdeau P, Kassab Chahmi D, Le Gal G, et al. 2008 SOR guidelines for the prevention and treatment of thrombosis associated with central venous

catheters in patients with cancer: report from the working group. *Ann Oncol.* 2009;20(9):1459-1471.

22. Kvale PA, Selecky PA, Prakash UB. Palliative care in lung cancer: ACCP evidence-based clinical practice guidelines (2nd ed.). *Chest.* 2007;132(suppl 3):368S-403.

23. Rowell NP, Gleeson FV. Steroids, radiotherapy, chemotherapy, and stents for superior vena caval obstruction in carcinoma of the bronchus: a systematic review. *Clin Oncol (R Coll Radiol).* 2002;14(5):338-351.

24. Uberoi R. Quality assurance guidelines for superior vena cava stenting in malignant disease. *Cardiovasc Intervent Radiol.* 2006;29(3):319-322.

25. Yoon HY, Cheon YK, Choi HJ, et al. Role of photodynamic therapy in the palliation of obstructing esophageal cancer. *Korean J Intern Med.* 2012;27(3):278-284.

26. Yu JB, Wilson LD, Detterbeck FC. Superior vena cava syndrome—a proposed classification system and algorithm for management. *J Thorac Oncol.* 2008;3(8):811-814.

27. Nagata T, Makutani S, Uchida H, et al. Follow-up results of 71 patients undergoing metallic stent placement for the treatment of a malignant obstruction of the superior vena cava. *Cardiovasc Intervent Radiol.* 2007;30(5):959-967.

28. Courtheoux P, Alkofer B, Al Refaï M, et al. Stent placement in superior vena cava syndrome. *Ann Thorac Surg.* 2003;75(1):158-161.

29. Lepper PM, Ott SR, Hoppe H, et al. Superior vena cava syndrome in thoracic malignancies. *Respir Care.* 2011;56(5):653-666.

30. Armstrong BA, Perez CA, Simpson JR, et al. Role of irradiation in the management of superior vena cava syndrome. *Int J Radiat Oncol Biol Phys.* 1987;13(4):531-539.

31. Gupta E. Palliative radiation therapy in superior vena cava obstruction in patients with advanced non-small cell lung cancer: a single institution experience. Presented at Kolkata, India 2012; 34th Annual Conference of the Association of Radiation Oncologists of India, AROICON 2012.

32. Lee HN, Tiwana MS, Saini M, et al. Superior vena cava obstruction (SVCO) in patients with advanced nonsmall cell lung cancer (NSCLC). *Gulf J Oncolog.* 2014;1(15):56-62.

33. Sundstrøm S, Bremnes R, Brunsvig P, et al. Immediate or delayed radiotherapy in advanced nonsmall cell lung cancer (NSCLC)? Data from a prospective randomised study. *Radiother Oncol.* 2005;75(2):141-148.

34. Falk SJ, Girling DJ, White RJ, et al. Immediate versus delayed palliative thoracic radiotherapy in patients with unresectable locally advanced non-small cell lung cancer and minimal thoracic symptoms: randomised controlled trial. *BMJ.* 2002;325(7362):465-468.

35. Pfister DG, Johnson DH, Azzoli CG, et al. American society of clinical oncology treatment of unresectable non-small-cell lung cancer guideline: update 2003. *J Clin Oncol.* 2004;22(24):330-353.

36. Davidoff AJ, Tang M, Seal B, et al. Chemotherapy and survival benefit in elderly patients with advanced non-small-cell lung cancer. *J Clin Oncol.* 2010;28(13):2191-2197.

37. Slotman B, van Tinteren H, Praag J, et al. Use of thoracic radiotherapy for extensive stage small-cell lung cancer: a phase 3 randomised controlled trial. *Lancet.* 2015;385(9962):36-42.

38. Lutz S, Chow E, Hartsell W, et al. A review of hypofractionated palliative radiotherapy. *Cancer.* 2007;109(8):1462-1470.

39. Wong J, Xu B, Yeung HN, et al. Age disparity in palliative radiation therapy among patients with advanced cancer. *Int J Radiat Oncol Biol Phys.* 2014;90(1):224-230.

40. Nieder C, Angelo K, Haukland E, et al. Survival after palliative radiotherapy in geriatric cancer patients. *Anticancer Res.* 2014;34(11):6641-6645.

41. Stevens R, Macbeth F, Toy E, et al. Palliative radiotherapy regimens for patients with thoracic symptoms from non-small cell lung cancer. *Cochrane Database Syst Rev.* 2015;1:CD002143.

42. Fairchild A, Harris K, Barnes E, et al. Palliative thoracic radiotherapy for lung cancer: a systematic review. *J Clin Oncol.* 2008;26(24):4001-4011.

43. Samant R, Gooi A. Radiotherapy basics for family physicians: potential tool for symptom relief. *Can Fam Physician.* 2005;51(11):1496-1501.

44. MRC Lung Cancer Working Party. Inoperable non–small cell lung cancer (NSCLC): a Medical Research Council randomized trial of palliative radiotherapy with two fractions or ten fractions. *Br J Cancer.* 1991;63(2):265-270.

45. MRC Lung Cancer Working Party. A Medical Research Council (MRC) randomised trial of palliative radiotherapy with two fractions or a single fraction in patients with inoperable non–small-cell lung cancer (NSCLC) and poor performance status. *Br J Cancer.* 1992;65(6):931-941.

46. Reuben DB, Mor V. Dyspnea in terminally ill cancer patients. *Chest.* 1986;89(2):234-236.

47. Kramer GW, Wanders SL, Noordijk EM, et al. Results of the Dutch national study of the palliative effect of irradiation using two different treatment schemes for non-small-cell lung cancer. *J Clin Oncol.* 2005;23(13):2962-2970.

48. MRC Lung Cancer Working Party. Randomized trial of palliative two-fraction versus more intensive 13-fraction radiotherapy for patients with inoperable non-small cell lung cancer and good performance status. *Clin Oncol (R Coll Radiol).* 1996;8(3):167-175.

49. Sundstrom S, Bremnes R, Aasebo U, et al. Hypofractionated palliative radiotherapy (17 Gy per 2 fractions) in advanced non-small cell lung carcinoma is comparable to standard fractionation for symptom control and survival: a national phase III trial. *J Clin Oncol.* 2004;22(5):801-810.

50. Duisters C, Beurskens H, Nijsten S, et al. Palliative chest irradiation in sitting position in patients with bulky advanced lung cancer. *Radiother Oncol.* 2006;79(3):285-287.

51. Marks LB, Yorke ED, Jackson A, et al. Use of normal tissue complication probability models in the clinic. *Int J Radiat Oncol Biol Phys*. 2010;76 (suppl 3):S10-19.

52. National Comprehensive Cancer Network. Non-small cell lung cancer (Version 1.2016). Available from http://www.nccn.org/professionals/ physician_gls/pdf/nscl.pdf. Accessed October 25, 2015.

53. Wang L, Yorke E, Desobry G, et al. Dosimetric advantage of using 6 MV over 15 MV photons in conformal therapy of lung cancer: Monte Carlo studies in patient geometries. *J Appl Clin Med Phys*. 2002;3(1):51-59.

54. Weiss E, Siebers JV, Keall PJ. An analysis of 6-MV versus 18-MV photon energy plans for intensity-modulated radiation therapy (IMRT) of lung cancer. *Radiother Oncol*. 2007;82(1):55-62.

55. Samant R, Gerig L, Montgomery L, et al. The emerging role of IG-IMRT for palliative radiotherapy: a single-institution experience. *Current Oncol*. 2009;16(3):40-45.

56. Topkan E, Yildirim BA, Guler OC, et al. Safety and palliative efficacy of single-dose 8 Gy reirradiation for painful local failure in patients with stage IV non-small cell lung cancer previously treated with radical chemoradiation therapy. *Int J Radiat Oncol Biol Phys*. 2015;91(4):774-780.

57. Griffioen GH, Dahele M, de Haan PF, et al. High-dose, conventionally fractionated thoracic reirradiation for lung tumors. *Lung Cancer*. 2014;83(3):356-362.

58. Drodge CS, Ghosh S, Fairchild A. Thoracic reirradiation for lung cancer: a literature review and practical guide. *Ann Palliat Med*. 2014;3(2):75-91.

59. Jeremic B, Videtic GM. Chest reirradiation with external beam radiotherapy for locally recurrent non-small-cell lung cancer: a review. *Int J Radiat Oncol Biol Phys*. 2011;80(4):969-977.

60. Rodrigues G, Macbeth F, Burmeister B, et al. Consensus statement on palliative lung radiotherapy: third international consensus workshop on palliative radiotherapy and symptom control. *Clin Lung Cancer*. 2012;13(1):1-5.

61. Dagnault A, Ebacher A, Vigneault E, et al. Retrospective study of 81 patients treated with brachytherapy for endobronchial primary tumor or metastasis. *Brachytherapy*. 2010;9(3):243-247.

62. Reveiz L, Rueda JR, Cardona AF. Palliative endobronchial brachytherapy for non-small cell lung cancer. *Cochrane Database Syst Rev*. 2012;12:004284.

63. Simoff MJ, Lally B, Slade MG, et al. Symptom management in patients with lung cancer: diagnosis and management of lung cancer, 3rd ed.: American College of Chest Physicians evidence-based clinical practice guidelines. *Chest*. 2013;143(suppl 5):455S-97S.

64. Ung YC, Yu E, Falkson C. The role of high-dose-rate brachytherapy in the palliation of symptoms in patients with non-small cell lung cancer: a systematic review. *Brachytherapy*. 2006;5(3):189-202.

65. Spiro S, Douse J, Read C, et al. Complications of lung cancer treatment. *Semin Respir Crit Care Med*. 2008;29(3):302-318.

66. Rorth M, Andersen C, Quist M, et al. Health benefits of a multidimensional exercise program for cancer patients undergoing chemotherapy. *Proc Am Soc Clin Oncol*. 2005;23(16S):731S.

67. Metcalfe S, Milano M, Bylund K, et al. Split-course palliative radiotherapy for advanced non-small cell lung cancer. *J Thor Oncol*. 2010;5(2):185-190.

68. Miranda V, Trufelli D, Santos J, et al. Effectivness of guarana (*Paullinia cupana*) for postradiation fatigue and depression: results of a pilot double-blind randomized study. *J Altern Complement Med*. 2009;15(4):431-433.

69. Tanner C. Palliative radiation therapy for cancer. *J Pall Med*. 2011;14(5):672-673.

70. Kassam Z, Wong R, Ringash J, et al. A phase I/II study to evaluate the toxicity and efficacy of accelerated fractionation radiotherapy for the palliation of dysphagia from carcinoma of the esophagus. *Clin Oncol (R Coll Radiol)*. 2008;20(1):53-60.

71. Howell D. The role of radiation therapy in the palliation of gastrointestinal malignancies. *Gastroenterol Clin N Am*. 2006; 35(1): 125-130.

8 Abdominal and Pelvic Malignancies

Sushmita Ghoshal, Bhavana Rai, and Raviteja Miriyala

INTRODUCTION

Radiation oncologists have long understood the potential benefit of radiation therapy (RT) in palliating the distressing symptoms of advanced abdominal and pelvic cancers. Often, the role of external beam radiation therapy (EBRT) or brachytherapy in controlling bleeding or obstructive symptoms finds only a passing reference[1] and most palliative medicine texts are silent on this important topic. Apprehension of radiation-induced toxicities may be one reason for this omission. This argument is not entirely valid, as various short course palliative radiation schedules are planned such that treatment-related acute toxicity is minimal. Because the majority of patients treated with palliative intent have limited life expectancies, treatment-related late toxicity is seldom a major concern; moreover, it is important to weigh the potential toxicity against the efficacy and improvement in a patient's quality of life (QoL).

Carcinomas arising in intra-abdominal organs are generally not treated with curative intent with RT alone due to a lack of therapeutic benefit. However, patients with advanced, inoperable disease may obtain symptom relief when treated by a short course of radiation. Intraluminal brachytherapy has been used for palliating obstructive symptoms of biliary tract cancers[2] and is a safe procedure with minimal morbidity.[3] Palliative RT achieves hemostasis in patients with unresectable gastric carcinoma not fit for systemic chemotherapy[4] and is associated with a statistically significant rise in their hemoglobin levels. Several other studies have confirmed this benefit though the doses of radiation varied from a single fraction of 8 to 50 Gy in 25 fractions. All dose schemes have benefits in symptom control, with no statistically significant differences between patients who received a biologically effective dose (BED) less or more than 39 Gy, assuming the alpha-beta ratio to be 10.[5]

EBRT is an integral part of multimodality treatment for carcinoma of the rectum and anal canal and provides relief to patients with locally advanced or recurrent disease not amenable to surgical excision.[6] Pelvis masses can cause pain, obstruction, tenesmus, bleeding, and discharge. Though most studies are retrospective without patient-reported QoL, they consistently demonstrate symptom relief and improved QoL with palliative pelvic RT. No statistically significant dose–response relationship has been established. James et al. reported a similar median duration of response in patients receiving <15 Gy or more.[7] In the systematic review of palliative RT by Cameron et al[8] in incurable primary and recurrent rectal cancer by palliative EBRT, all of the 27 studies reported good relief of pain, bleeding, and mass effect with acceptable toxicities. None of these studies had patient reported outcomes and various dose-fractionations were used. Most of these studies were retrospective chart reviews of patients treated more than two decades ago, with incomplete follow up. Despite these inherent shortcomings, the pooled response to palliative pelvic EBRT ranged from 71% to 81%. It was not possible to calculate the BED for comparison of different dose schedules. There is a need for prospective studies using modern RT techniques and uniform endpoints, to provide robust evidence about the risk–benefit ratio of palliative pelvic RT in advanced rectal carcinoma. In patients with locally advanced and metastatic rectal cancer,[35] a hypofractionated radiation therapy course can limit the need for palliative colostomy to 33%. This regimen was associated with an 82% local control rate with less than 10% mild acute toxicity and no late toxicity.

Patients with locally advanced or metastatic bladder cancer may benefit from palliative RT to the pelvis. Fossa and Hosbach reported on their experience treating all symptomatic patients above age 80 and younger patients with distant metastasis with palliative pelvic RT.[9] Using a moderate dose of 30 Gy in 10 fractions over 2 weeks, patients experienced a significant reduction in hematuria. In a retrospective review of 94 patients, Salminen reported complete and partial relief of symptoms, 43% and 29% respectively, with 30 Gy in 6 fractions over 3 weeks.[10] Eight out of 17 patients did not need the indwelling catheter after radiation. The estimated median survival was 9.6 months. There was a local control rate of 40% which was associated with longer survival. In a systematic overview article, Widmark et al. reported that it is possible to decrease tumor-induced bladder symptoms rapidly and effectively with palliative EBRT.[11] Also, a hypofractionated 1-week regimen was as effective as a 2-week daily treatment in doing this.

RT has been used for symptom relief in gynecological malignancies for many years. Both brachytherapy and EBRT have been used successfully to obtain hemostasis in carcinoma cervix. Boulware et al., from the MD Anderson Cancer Center, published their experience using hypofractionated radiation 10 Gy once a month for 3 months.[12] After 3 fractions, vaginal bleeding was controlled in all patients. However, care must be taken to not to use very high doses per fraction radiation for patients with potentially curable disease and long anticipated survival. In addition to bleeding, radiation palliates pain, obstructive symptoms, and vaginal discharge. Sklirenko and Barnes reported overall symptom response rates of 45% to 100% for bleeding, 0% to 83% for pain, 39% to 49% for discharge, and 19% to 100% for obstructive symptoms.[13] The RTOG 7905 trial was based on the MD Anderson experience and added concurrent Misonidazole, a hypoxic cell sensitizer, to the radiation. This trial closed prematurely due to excessive gastrointestinal complications and a different hypofractionated regimen was designed.[14] RTOG 8502, used twice a day radiation for 2 days, 3.7 Gy/fraction, a regimen now known as the QUAD shot. The cycle was repeated monthly up to a maximum of three times or maximum dose of 44.4 Gy.[15,16] This led to a significant decrease in early and late toxicities. At Princess Margaret Hospital (PMH), 7 Gy/fraction is delivered on a weekly basis for 3 weeks.[17] In their 10-year experience, vaginal bleeding was controlled in 92% patients and the regimen was comparable to the other hypofractionated regimens in terms of efficacy and toxicity.

Two centers in India who routinely use monthly palliative pelvic radiation for advanced carcinoma cervix published their experience of using parallel opposed megavoltage radiation. Mishra et al. used 10 Gy/fraction[18] with additional brachytherapy in five patients while Rai et al.[19] used 8 Gy/fraction. Both studies reported good control of symptoms like vaginal bleeding, discharge, and pain. Carcinoma of the cervix is a common disease within developing countries, where many patients report late to the hospital with incurable disease. A short course of hypofractionated radiation can control their distressing symptoms, improve QoL, and reduce hospitalization with minimal treatment-related toxicity.

It is unlikely that prolonged fractionation can produce more effective or durable palliation as compared to short, hypofractionated ones. Since higher radiation doses per fraction have a higher potential for late toxicity, which generally occurs 9 months after completion of treatment. Therefore, it is important to carefully select patients for hypofractionation. In patients with limited life expectancies, a short but effective dose of palliative pelvic radiation will produce adequate symptom relief without increasing the burden for patients and caregivers.

TREATMENT PLANNING BY SITE

The aim of palliative RT is to improve the QoL of patients with incurable disease, by providing maximum symptom relief, while minimizing treatment-related acute toxicities and durations of hospital stays. This can be achieved by minimizing the field sizes and number of fractions while maintaining the therapeutic index.

With proper patient selection, delayed toxicities are seldom of concern while planning palliative RT, thereby allowing a wider freedom in choosing the field sizes and target volumes for various sites. Hence, it becomes impractical to have stringent practice guidelines for planning palliative RT. Treatment planning recommendations for typical case scenarios encountered in clinical practice are given in the following section. However, treatment volumes and field sizes should be selected appropriately on a patient-by-patient basis, considering various factors like life expectancy, performance status, disease burden, severity of symptoms, comorbidities, goals of therapy, and departmental logistics.

Most often, conventional planning based on bony landmarks is adequate for treatment planning, especially in developing countries with limited resources. In centers where conventional simulators have been superseded by CT simulators, virtual simulation is used for treatment planning.

The following cases illustrate the role of palliative-radiation therapy in the treatment of bladder cancer, vaginal bleeding, rectal cancer, vulvar cancer, and liver metastasis. Further discussion of the role of palliative radiation therapy for liver tumors can be found in Chapter 9.

Case 8.1: Palliative Treatment of the Bladder

A 75-year-old patient of carcinoma of the urinary bladder, with widespread bone and lung metastases, presents with dysuria and pelvic pain. He had coronary artery disease and a poor performance status. Being unsuitable for systemic chemotherapy, he was planned for palliative pelvic RT.

Simulation for such patients is done in the supine position, preferably with an empty bladder. Parallel opposed antero-posterior fields are generally used. The upper border is placed at L5–S1 interface; lower border at the level of ischial tuberosities; lateral borders are placed 2-cm lateral to the widest part of the pelvic brim (Figure 8.1).

If virtual simulation is planned, a noncontrast CT scan is taken in supine position with empty bladder. Gross tumor along with the entire urinary bladder and prostatic urethra is delineated and a margin (2–2.5 cm) is given to account for internal motion and set up uncertainties. Conformal radiation with two or three fields is delivered using multileaf collimation (Figure 8.2).

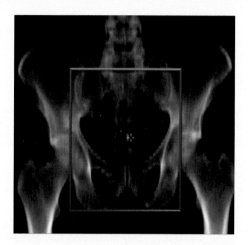

FIGURE 8.1 Palliative RT portal for antero-posterior fields, urinary bladder cancer.

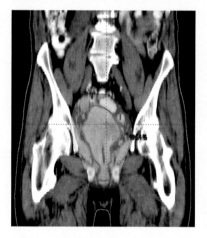

FIGURE 8.2 Conformal radiation plan for urinary bladder cancer.

Case 8.2: Palliative Radiation for Vaginal Bleeding

A 68-year-old female presented with foul smelling discharge and bleeding *per vaginum*; examination revealed a large ulcero-proliferative growth replacing the entire cervix and extending to the lateral pelvic walls, with a frozen pelvis. After further evaluation she was diagnosed with poorly differentiated squamous cell cancer of the cervix, with extensive para-aortic and supraclavicular nodal metastases, and bilateral gross hydro-uretero-nephrosis and deranged renal function. She was planned for palliative pelvic radiation.

For such patients, a four-field box technique or a simpler two-field technique is adequate for palliation. Simulation is done in supine position with an empty bladder. Simple positioning devices like knee wedges may be used. The upper margin of the field is generally placed at L4–L5 interface; however, it can be brought down to L5–S1 interface in certain cases if field size is too large. Lateral margins are placed 2-cm lateral to the widest part of the pelvic brim. Lower margin should be placed at least 2 cm beyond the lower extent of the disease, and inferior margin of the obturator foramen is an adequate bony landmark for most cases (Figure 8.3). However, if there is extension of growth into the lower vagina, the patient should be simulated in a frog-leg position with antero-posterior fields, and lower border placed to cover the introitus. For patients without lower vaginal extension, two lateral fields can be added by placing the anterior border at the anterior

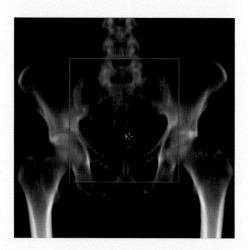

FIGURE 8.3 Antero-posterior portals for palliative RT of cervical cancer.

cortex of pubic symphysis and posterior border to cover the sacral hollow (Figure 8.4). Virtual simulation and conformal planning may be used in selected cases and fields with differential weightage can be used for improved dose distribution.

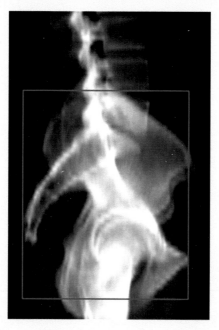

FIGURE 8.4 Lateral fields for palliative RT of cervical cancer.

Case 8.3: Palliative Radiation Therapy for Rectal Cancer

A 65-year-old patient with adenocarcinoma of the rectum underwent abdomino-perineal resection and adjuvant chemotherapy 7 years ago. Now he presented with multiple liver metastases, along with local recurrence, causing pelvic pain. He did not respond to second-line chemotherapy, and was offered palliative pelvic RT.

Simulation for patients of rectal cancer is generally done in the prone position for better reproducibility, unless patients have an existing colostomy. Antero-posterior fields or four-field box technique is generally used, similar to patients of cervical cancer; however, the upper margins are usually placed at L5–S1 interface. For lateral fields, the anterior margins are placed at the posterior cortex of symphysis pubis, and posterior border is generally placed 1.5 cm behind the anterior sacral margin (Figure 8.5). For conformal radiation, gross primary tumor along with adequate margins on either side is delineated and a margin is given for set up errors. Generally, uninvolved nodal regions are not included in palliative radiation.

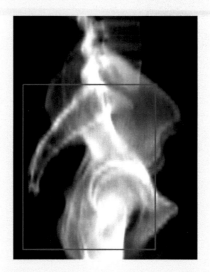

FIGURE 8.5 Lateral portals for four-field box technique, rectal cancer.

Case 8.4: Palliative Radiation Therapy for Vulvar Cancer

A 73-year-old female presented with a large ulcero-proliferative growth over her external genitalia, and was diagnosed as a case of vulval cancer, extending into the lower third of vagina and urethra. Due to multiple comorbidities and poor performance status, she was considered for palliative RT.

Simulation for such patients of vulval cancer is preferably done in frog-leg position, and antero-posterior fields are adequate. Tissue equivalent bolus material is generally placed during treatment to increase the superficial dose. Upper border is placed at midsacroiliac joint and lower border should flash the entire perineum and the gross disease with adequate margin. Lateral borders are placed 2-cm lateral to the pelvic inlet. If there is gross inguinal nodal enlargement, fields may be extended laterally. Alternatively, a single incident field may be used by rotating the couch and gantry for treating the gross disease in appropriately selected patients (Figure 8.6).

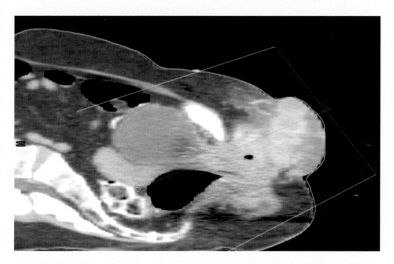

FIGURE 8.6 Single-field technique with couch and gantry rotation for palliation of vulval cancer.

Case 8.5: Palliative Radiation Therapy to the Liver

A 56-year-old male patient was diagnosed as a case of pancreatic cancer with multiple liver metastases. Response to systemic chemotherapy was suboptimal; a biliary stent was placed to relieve obstructive symptoms but the patient had persistent pain in the upper abdomen radiating to the back. He was planned for palliative RT.

For abdominal malignancies, bony landmarks are less reliable for treatment planning, as compared to pelvic malignancies. For such patients, virtual simulation on a plain or contrast-enhanced CT scan is preferable to ensure adequate coverage. Gross primary disease responsible for the symptoms is delineated and a margin is given for uncertainties. Elective nodal irradiation is not generally indicated (Figure 8.7). If CT simulation is not available, wide antero-posterior fields extending between D11 and L2 vertebral bodies are used, and lateral margins are placed according to the location and extent of the disease, with renal shielding in appropriate cases.

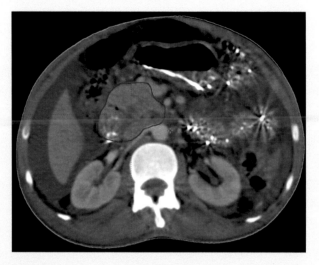

FIGURE 8.7 Delineation of gross tumor in pancreatic cancer for palliative radiation.

TOXICITY

Radiation-induced toxicities can be subdivided into acute, which occurs during or immediately after therapy, and late, which occurs several months after completion of treatment. Acute reactions depend on the total dose, dose per fraction, and overall treatment time while late reactions primarily depend on dose per fraction. A more modest total dose of RT and the limited life expectancy of the patient typically balance risk associated with the higher dose per fraction. Careful patient selection also minimizes the risk; hypofractionated RT with large RT dose per fraction should be used sparingly in frail patients with potentially curative disease who may live long enough to be at risk for late toxicity. Much of the available literature on palliative EBRT is retrospective with inadequate follow-up and toxicity data. In addition, it may be difficult to distinguish some of the late toxicities like fistula formation from disease progression. With the advent of modern radiation techniques delivering conformal therapy, normal tissues can be saved from unwanted radiation, which should reduce both acute and late toxicities.

The acute side effects of radiation include nausea, vomiting, anorexia, and fatigue. When the pelvis is irradiated, patients also complain of bowel and bladder symptoms. Salminen et al. reported that 62% of the bladder cancer patients experienced diarrhea. Sixteen percent of patients had severe acute toxicity[10] which resulted in treatment termination (5%) or interruption (7%). Urinary frequency or incontinence was found in 20% of patients. The use of two anterior-posterior fields was associated with more severe toxicities than three or four field RT. Late effects, such as urethral stricture, proctitis, cystitis, small bowel injury, and urinary incontinence, were noted in 29% of patients more than 3 months after completion of treatment. The incidence of late effects was significantly higher in patients with longer field size. There were no treatment-related deaths in the group of patients studied.

Skliarenko and Barnes evaluated the role of pelvic RT for gynecological cancers and reported an overall late toxicity rate of 6% to 12% occurring 9 to 10 months after treatment.[13] To reduce the risk of severe late toxicities, the third fraction of 10 Gy could be omitted if adequate symptom relief was achieved by two fractions. The RTOG 7905 reported excessively high late GI toxicities because of the radiation sensitizer Misonidazole.[14] Their subsequent trial 8502 showed a marked reduction in late toxicity—only 6% late complications were noted.[15,16] Among the 51 patients treated by the PMH group,[17] only two complained of severe late toxicities.

Kim et al.[20] used short course palliative radiation for cancers of the uterine cervix. Using three-dimensional conformal radiation, they delivered 20 to 25 Gy with 5 Gy/fraction. Only 7 of 17 patients had minor gastrointestinal toxicity and one patient had grade three diarrhea 1 week after treatment. Late complications were seen in four patients but none had grade three or higher severity. Hypofractionated, conformal pelvic radiation is likely to be effective and less toxic but more randomized, prospective trials are required to establish these facts. The life expectancy of the patient should always be considered when selecting appropriate fractionation schedules.

SYMPTOM MANAGEMENT

Recurrent and advanced abdominal and pelvic malignancies can cause severely distressing symptoms resulting in a poor QoL. Effective palliation of these symptoms can often be achieved using uncomplicated treatment practices with minimal morbidity and treatment decisions should be based on improving the QoL. Depending on the site and patterns of spread, the symptoms may vary from patient to patient. The most common symptoms include bleeding, pain, discharge, urinary/bowel fistulas, obstruction, lower extremity edema, deep vein thrombosis, fungating wounds, and ascites.

For a patient presenting with bleeding, it is important to first identify the cause. Bleeding may occur due to tumor infiltration of the blood vessels, systemic complications such as thrombocytopenia and underlying coagulopathy, use of drugs such as nonsteroidal anti-inflammatory drugs (NSAIDs) and anticoagulants, and concurrent illness including infection.

The patient presenting with acute hemorrhage should be put on bed rest and hemodynamic support along with administration of anxiolytics and/or sedatives. Rapid acting sedatives such as intravenous or subcutaneous midazolam 2.5 or 5 mg should be administered and may be repeated if necessary. Drugs like oral tranexamic acid have been found to be helpful in patients with mild bleeds but need to be used cautiously in cases of bleeding from the bladder due to risk of clot retention. For patients with vaginal bleeding, tight vaginal packing is very useful in cases of acute hemorrhage. Depending on the institutional practice, the pack may be soaked in povidone-iodine, acriflavin, or thrombostatic agents. The vaginal pack is usually left in situ for 24 to 48 hours, during which the patient can be hemodynamically stabilized and planned for palliative external RT or brachytherapy.[21,22] Repeated vaginal packing should be done if required. Large doses of hypofractionated RT have been found to be extremely effective in controlling vaginal and rectal bleeds, bleeds from fungating ulcers, and hematuria. The cessation of bleeding usually occurs in 12 to 48 hours after treatment. Although a number of fractionation schedules have been used, there is at present no evidence that protracted radiation results in more effectual palliation.[23,24] Dose per fraction of 8 to 10 Gy as a single fraction or 2 to 3 fractions repeated at monthly intervals have not only resulted in effective symptom control, but are also cost-effective and logistically suitable to the already distressed patient and the care givers.[25]

Transcutaneous arterial embolization (TAE) may be considered in selected patients in whom noninvasive measures and radiation fail to control bleeding. Occasionally, it may also be used upfront in cases of massive hemorrhage. The procedure involves embolization of the iliac vessels using coils, gel foam, and so on. The evidence regarding its use in the palliative setting is largely based on case reports and short series. Thus, arterial embolization should be attempted only in a suitable patient where the facilities for the same are available.

Symptoms such as pain, pressure symptoms due to soft-tissue masses, and bony invasion by tumor are managed with analgesics and adjuvant drugs according to the World Health Organization (WHO) step ladder pattern, depending on the type and severity of the symptoms. RT has been found to be very effective in providing a relatively sustained relief of these symptoms. While the majority of studies in this regard are limited to cervical cancer, the results of the same may be extrapolated to other sites in the pelvis. Relief of pain has been reported in 40% and 100% of patients in various studies with stabilization of pain reported in nearly 50% of patients.[8,18,19] Similarly, relief of obstructive symptoms in patients with advanced rectal cancers has been reported in nearly two-thirds of patients receiving palliative pelvic RT with 1/3rd reporting symptom control at 1 year after treatment.[8,26] Vaginal discharge or discharge from the rectum can be a very distressing symptom. The few studies evaluating the role of RT have reported in a wide variation in response ranging from 15% to 100%.[18,27] In addition, significant relief dysuria, obstipation, and tenesmus have been observed with RT.[28]

Although palliative RT along with appropriate medical management plays a pivotal role in symptom management of advanced incurable cancers, it needs to be cautiously administered in patients with disease-related fistulas as it may lead to exacerbation of symptoms and a deterioration in QoL. Terminally ill patients presenting with uremia and obstructive uropathy should be managed with best supportive care. The decision to perform an invasive per cutaneous nephrostomy should be individualized and its role in very advanced/recurrent/residual disease seems controversial. Though the procedure may transiently improved renal function, it typically only prolongs the patient's pain and suffering. In such cases, prolonging survival by preventing death from uremia may come with the price of reduced QoL because of pain, fatigue, recurrent infections, or other sequel of advanced metastatic disease.[29]

Patients with advanced abdominal malignancies usually present with upper gastro-intestinal bleeding, pain, biliary obstruction, and ascites. Although the medical management is essentially similar, RT has a relatively limited role in management of hemorrhage in these patients, especially with the evolution of advanced endoscopic techniques that can effectively control hemorrhage.[30] For pain management, apart from the standard WHO step ladder, percutaneous celiac plexus blockage may benefit patients with poor response to or poor tolerance of opioid analgesics.[31] Radiation can be considered as an alternative treatment in management of poorly controlled pain in advanced pancreatic cancers. Jaundice with associated pruritus, malaise, loss of appetite, and abdominal discomfort commonly occur in patients with advanced pancreatic cancers. Percutaneous transhepatic biliary drainage or endoscopic stent placement provides an excellent outcome in these patients.[32] Those with malignant bowel obstruction are best managed conservatively with a combination of metoclopramide, octreotide, and steroids given in appropriate doses. In patients with advanced gastric cancers, symptoms like intractable vomiting due to gastric outlet obstruction can be relieved by proximal decompression using nasogastric tube insertion, percutaneous endoscopic gastrostomy (PEG), or gastric stenting.[33,34] In addition, patients with advanced pelvic and abdominal cancers often present with symptoms of ascites and deep vein thrombosis. For ascites, a combination of repeated therapeutic paracentesis and diuretic therapy or peritoneo-venous shunts helps ameliorate the discomfort. Management of deep vein thrombosis can be challenging as these patients are also at a risk of bleeding. The recommended management includes the use of low-molecular-weight heparins. The aim of management in patients with advanced incurable cancers should be enhancement of QoL, even though the survival is limited.

CLINICAL PEARLS

- RT is an effective modality for palliation of symptoms due to pelvic malignancies, like pain, bleeding, or discharge.
- Availability of alternative modalities using endoscopic techniques, along with inherent lack of favorable therapeutic benefit, limits the role of radiation therapy for palliation of abdominal malignancies.
- Optimal patient selection after considering various factors like severity of symptoms, disease burden, performance status, life expectancy, patient convenience, and departmental logistics, is paramount for deciding on the fractionation schedule.
- Single or limited fractions of higher doses of radiation are often preferred for patients with limited life expectancies.
- Various short course fractionated regimens have been developed for patients with longer life expectancies, to optimally balance the treatment duration and probability of radiation-induced late effects.
- Optimal utilization of available resources, along with appropriate supportive care by a multidisciplinary team, is necessary for improving the QoL of patients with pelvic and abdominal malignancies.

SELF-ASSESSMENT

Questions

1. The preferred modality for controlling hematemesis in a patient of metastatic gastric cancer is
   A. External RT
   B. Endoscopic hemostasis
   C. Chemotherapy
   D. Targeted therapy

2. Choose the false statement among the following, regarding biliary tract cancer.
   A. Percutaneous transhepatic biliary drainage is an accepted modality for relieving obstructive symptoms
   B. Brachytherapy is never used for palliation

    C. SBRT has a limited role in management of inoperable gall bladder cancer

    D. Repeated paracentesis can be done to relieve malignant ascites

3. In a male patient with metastatic urinary bladder cancer, the treatment portals for palliative RT should include all of the following, except
    A. Dome of the bladder
    B. Neck of the bladder
    C. Prostatic urethra
    D. Inguinal lymph nodes

4. All of the following can be used for controlling vaginal bleeding in a palliative patient of cervical cancer, except
    A. Vaginal packing
    B. Tranexemic acid
    C. External radiation
    D. Radiofrequency ablation

5. The best modality for management of pelvic pain in a patient with inoperable metastatic rectal cancer is
    A. Chemotherapy
    B. Cetuximab
    C. External RT
    D. Trans arterial embolization

6. A relative contraindication for palliative RT in a patient with vulval cancer is
    A. Bleeding
    B. Discharge
    C. Ulceration
    D. Vescico-vaginal fistula

Answers

1. B. For an overtly bleeding vessel causing hematemesis, endoscopic treatment results in more immediate hemostasis. Radiation therapy is more useful in oozing in the absence of an identifiable vessel. Radiation therapy has been reported to control hematemesis and improve hemoglobin levels but the series are small.

2. B. Intraluminal brachytherapy palliates obstructive symptoms of biliary tract cancers. EBRT has also been used with minimal morbidity.

3. D. Inguinal lymph nodes are rarely the cause of symptoms in bladder cancer. To palliate bladder cancer, the entire bladder should be in the target volume.

4. D. Radiation therapy, vaginal packing, and administration of tranexamic acid are viable treatment options for vaginal bleeding. Radiofrequency ablation has not been used in this setting.

5. C. Radiation therapy effectively palliates pelvic pain due to locally advanced rectal cancer with response rates of 70% to 80%.

6. D. Bleeding, discharge, and ulceration can be effectively palliated with EBRT. A vesico-vaginal fistula cannot be palliated with radiation therapy.

REFERENCES

1. Halperin EC, Brady LW, Perez CA, Wazer DE. *Perez & Brady's Principles and Practice of Radiation Oncology*. Philadelphia, PA: Lippincott Williams & Wilkins, 2013.
2. Gonzalez D, Gouma DJ, Rauws EA, et al. Role of radiotherapy, in particular intraluminal brachytherapy, in the treatment of proximal bile duct carcinoma. *Ann Oncol*. 1999;10(4):215-220.
3. Houry S, Haccart V, Huguier M, et al. Gallbladder cancer: role of radiation therapy. *Hepatogastroenterology*. 1999;46:1578-1584.
4. Chaw CL, Niblock PG, Chaw CS, et al. The role of palliative radiotherapy for haemostasis in unresectable gastric cancer: a single-institution experience. *Ecancermedicalscience*. 2014;8:384.
5. Tey J, Back MF, Shakespeare TP, et al. The role of palliative radiation therapy in symptomatic locally advanced gastric cancer. *Int J Radiat Oncol Biol Phys*. 2007;67:385-388.
6. Wong R, Thomas G, Cummings B, et al. The role of radiotherapy in the management of pelvic recurrence of rectal cancer. *Can J Oncol*. 1996;6(1):39-47.
7. James RD, Johnson RJ, Eddleston B, et al. Prognostic factors in locally recurrent rectal carcinoma treated by radiotherapy. *Br J Surg*. 1983;70:469-472.
8. Cameron MG, Kersten C, Vistad I, et al. Palliative pelvic radiotherapy of symptomatic incurable rectal cancer: a systematic review. *Acta Oncol*. 2014;53(2):164-173.
9. Fosså SD, Hosbach G. Short-term moderate-dose pelvic radiotherapy of advanced bladder carcinoma. A questionnaire-based evaluation of its symptomatic effect. *Acta Oncol*. 1991;30(6):735-738.
10. Salminen E. Unconventional fractionation for palliative radiotherapy of urinary bladder cancer: a retrospective review of 94 patients. *Acta Oncol*. 1992;31(4):449-454.
11. Widmark A, Flodgren P, Damber JE, et al. A systematic overview of radiation therapy effects in urinary bladder cancer. *Acta Oncol*. 2003;42(5):567-581.

12. Boulware RJ, Caderao JB, Declos L, et al. Whole pelvis megavoltage irradiation with single dose of 1000 rad to palliate advanced gynaecologic cancers. *Int J Radiat Oncol Biol Phys*. 1979;5:333-338.

13. Skliarenko J, Barnes EA. Palliative pelvic radiotherapy for gynaecologic cancer. *J Radiat Oncol*. 2012;1(3):239-244.

14. Spanos WJ Jr, Wasserman T, Meoz R, et al. Palliation of advanced pelvic malignant disease with large fraction pelvic radiation & misonidazole: final report on RTOG Phase-I/II study. *Int J Radiat Oncol Biol Phys*. 1987;13:1479-1482.

15. Spanos W Jr, Guse C, Perez C, et al. Phase II study of multiple daily fractionations in the palliation of advanced pelvic malignancies: preliminary report of RTOG 8502. *Int J Radiat Oncol Bio Phys*. 1989;17(3):659-661.

16. Spanos WJ Jr, Clery M, Perez CA. Late effect of multiple daily fraction palliation schedule for advanced pelvic malignancies (RTOG 8502). *Int J Radiat Oncol Biol Phys*. 1994;29(5):961-967.

17. Yan J, Milosevic M, Fyles A, et al. A hypofractionated radiotherapy regimen (0-7-21) for advanced gynaecological cancer patients. *Clin Oncol (R Coll Radiol)*. 2011;23(7):476-481.

18. Mishra SK, Laskar S, Muckaden MA, et al. Monthly palliative pelvic radiotherapy in advanced carcinoma of uterine cervix. *J Cancer Res Ther*. 2005;1(4):208.

19. Rai B, Khosla D, Patel F, et al. Palliative radiotherapy in advanced cancer of the cervix. *Internet J Pain Symptom Control Palliat Care*. 2012;9(1).

20. Kim DH, Lee JH, Ki YK, et al. Short-course palliative radiotherapy for uterine cervical cancer. *Radiat Oncol J*. 2013;31(4):216-221.

21. Hulme B, Wilcox S. *Guidelines on the Management of Bleeding for Palliative Care Patients With Cancer*. On behalf of the Yorkshire Palliative Medicine Clinical Guidelines Group, 2008.

22. Lutz S, Chow E, Hoskin P. *Radiation Oncology in Palliative Cancer Care*. Hoboken, NJ: John Wiley & Sons, 2013.

23. May LF, Belinson JL, Roland TA. Palliative benefit of radiation therapy in advanced ovarian cancer. *Gynecol Oncol*. 1990;37(3):408-411.

24. Duchesne GM, Bolger JJ, Griffiths GO, et al. A randomized trial of hypofractionated schedules of palliative radiotherapy in the management of bladder carcinoma: results of medical research council trial BA09. *Int J Radiat Oncol Biol Phys*. 2000;47(2):379-388.

25. Lutz ST, Chow EL, Hartsell WF, Konski AA. A review of hypofractionated palliative radiotherapy. *Cancer*. 2007;109(8):1462-1470.

26. Bae SH, Park W, Choi DH, et al. Palliative radiotherapy in patients with a symptomatic pelvic mass of metastatic colorectal cancer. *Radiat Oncol*. 2011;6(1):1.

27. Onsrud M, Hagen B, Strickert T. 10 Gy single-fraction pelvic irradiation for palliation and life prolongation in patients with cancer of the cervix and corpus uteri. *Gynecol Oncol*. 2001;82:167-171.

28. Spanos Jr WJ, Pajak TJ, Emami B, et al. Radiation palliation of cervical cancer. *J Natl Cancer Inst Monogr*. 1996;2:127-130.

29. Keidan RD, Greenberg RE, Hoffman JP, Weese JL. Is percutaneous nephrostomy for hydronephrosis appropriate in patients with advanced cancer? *Am J Surg*. 1988;156(3):206-208.

30. Pereira J, Phan T. Management of bleeding in patients with advanced cancer. *Oncologist*. 2004;9(5):561-570.

31. Brescia FJ. Palliative care in pancreatic cancer. *Cancer Control*. 2004;11(1):39-45.

32. Boulay BR, Parepally M. Managing malignant biliary obstruction in pancreas cancer: choosing the appropriate strategy. *World J Gastroenterol*. 2014;20(28):9345-9353.

33. Blair SL, Chu DZ, Schwarz RE. Outcomes of palliative operations for malignant bowel obstruction in patients with peritoneal carcinomatosis from non gynecological cancer. *Ann Surg Oncol*. 2001;8:632-637.

34. Thaker DA, Stafford BC, Gaffney LS. Palliative management of malignant bowel obstruction in terminally ill patient. *Indian J Palliat Care*. 2010;16(2):97-100.

35. Janjan NA, Breslin T, Lenzi R, et al. Avoidance of colostomy placement in advanced colorectal cancer with twice weekly hypofractionated radiation plus continuous infusion 5-fluorouracil. *J Pain Symptom Manage*. 2000;20:266–272.

9   Liver Malignancies

Jared R. Robbins

INTRODUCTION

Each year in the United States there are estimated to be over 45,000 cases of primary liver and biliary system malignancies with over 28,000 deaths, and the incidence is rising.[1] Worldwide primary liver malignancies are the 6th most prevalent site of cancer, but in developing countries it is the 3rd most prevalent cancer.[2] Primary liver cancer exacts a significant toll on the worldwide population, causing over 700,000 deaths annually and is the third most common cause of cancer death overall, 2nd in men, and 6th in women.[3] While primary cancer is a major global health problem, secondary metastases to the liver are more common. Liver is the primary site of metastases for many malignant neoplasms, particularly those of the gastrointestinal (GI) tract because their draining blood supply is funneled into the portal venous system. Colorectal cancer is the third most common malignancy in the United States, the second leading cause of cancer death, and represents the majority of liver metastases. It is estimated that in 2015 there will be greater than 130,000 new cases of colorectal cancer in the United States.[1] Some estimate that 50% to 70% of patients with locally advanced colorectal cancer will eventually develop liver metastases. Aside from cancers of the GI tract (colorectal, stomach, pancreas, and esophagus), liver metastases frequently arise from lung cancer, breast cancer, and melanoma.

Patients with primary malignancy of the liver or liver metastases have relatively poor prognosis. The 5-year survival for primary liver cancers is less than 20%. Untreated hepatocellular carcinoma (HCC) has a median survival of 3 to 8.3 months.[4,5] Patients with limited disease that can be surgically treated may have improved long-term survival. The 5-year overall survival rate for individuals with early stage HCC who undergo liver transplants is 44% to 78%, while the 5-year survival for those undergoing liver resection is 27% to 70%.[6] Liver metastases also have poor prognoses, with patients with multiple liver metastases having a median survival of only a few months (2.5–7 months), but some patients with limited liver and systemic disease may have much longer survival after local therapies like surgery, liver ablation, or stereotactic body radiation therapy (SBRT).[7-12]

Although primary liver malignancies or metastases may be asymptomatic for some time after development, eventually untreated or recurrent disease in the liver will result in significant morbidity and symptoms. These can include abdominal pain, feeling of poor health or weakness, loss of appetite, weight loss, nausea/vomiting, fever, fatigue, bloating, abdominal distention, itching, lower extremity edema, jaundice, and liver failure. A summary of the frequency of the various symptoms can be seen in Table 9.1.

The four most common tumor types that require palliative liver treatments are HCC, cholangiocarcinoma, metastatic colorectal carcinoma, and metastatic neuroendocrine tumors.[2,15] While each may have slightly different presentations and symptoms secondary to differences in location, natural history, and histology, all have similar options for palliative treatments. Palliative methods for managing symptoms from advanced liver tumors including resection, ablation, vascular intervention, stenting, chemotherapy, medical management, and radiation therapy.[15] The proper application of each intervention varies somewhat by both patient-related and tumor-related factors. Appropriate selection of the most useful intervention is outside the scope of this chapter, but when possible, discussion in a multidisciplinary team (surgeons, interventional radiologists, medical oncologists, radiation oncologists, palliative care specialists) can help facilitate the most appropriate action for each patient. The purpose of this chapter is to discuss the use of external beam radiation therapy for palliation of liver malignancy and will focus primarily on external beam radiation therapy, but will also briefly discuss the use of SBRT and radioembolization.

In the early days of external beam radiation therapy with both cobalt units and newly minted linear accelerators, various groups started using whole liver external beam techniques (WLRT) to palliate symptomatic liver metastases. In the 1950s to 1970s, several groups published their retrospective institutional experiences.[9,10,16-19] These initial pioneering efforts showed great promise with effective palliation in the majority of patients with a reasonable toxicity profiles, with WLRT doses ranging from around 19 Gy to 31 Gy delivered in 2.5 to 4 weeks courses.[9,10,16-19] They also realized the sensitivity of the liver to whole

TABLE 9.1 Frequency of Symptoms Associated With Advanced or Refractory Primary and Secondary Liver Malignancies

Study	Abdominal Distention/ Ascites	Fatigue	Nausea	Night Sweats	Vomiting	Abdominal Pain	Anorexia	Jaundice
Borgelt[8]	48%	79%	34%	21%		76%	63%	29%
Bydder[13]	67%		64%	43%	29%	39%		
Soliman[14]	15%	7%	5%		15%	66%		

liver radiation doses of more than 30 Gy, which could result in radiation-induced hepatitis or radiation-induced liver disease (RILD).[17]

Building on the enthusiasm of these early experiences, the first multi-institutional trial evaluating the use of WLRT for the palliation of malignant liver disease was performed by the Radiation Therapy Oncology Group (RTOG 76-05). Incidentally, this was also the first RTOG study of a GI site, perhaps emphasizing the burden of symptomatic liver metastases at that time. This was a prospective, uncontrolled, nonrandomized pilot study designed to test the feasibility of hepatic irradiation for symptomatic metastatic liver disease using six separate radiation schemas (two for solitary metastases and four for multiple hepatic lesions or patients with metastatic disease outside of the liver). The regimens for solitary metastases included the initial whole liver fields followed by an optional boost to the solitary lesion up to 1/3 of the liver, while patients with multiple hepatic metastases were treating to the whole liver only. Specific details about the radiation therapy (RT) can be found in Table 9.2. Seventy-seven percent of the patients completed the treatment, while seven died prior to the completion of the RT. The median survival was 11 weeks. The most common side effect from the RT was nausea/vomiting in 16%. No patient developed radiation hepatitis, nephritis, or pneumonitis. Eight specific signs and symptoms were evaluated at 4 weeks post-treatment, and improvements were seen in all symptoms with the best responses for abdominal pain (55%), nausea/vomiting (49%), and fever/night sweats (45%). Complete responses for symptoms ranged from 7% (weakness/fatigue) to 34% (nausea/vomiting). Response rates were highest for those with the most symptomatic disease. Karnofsky performance status improved in 25% of patients and liver function improved in 37% to 48% of patients who presented with abnormal values. Overall, the authors estimated that patients with mild or no symptoms spent an average of 80% of their remaining lives with mild to no pain, while those with moderate or severe pain before treatment spent an average of 63% of their remaining lives with either mild or no pain.[8] Overall, this study was viewed as a success and was a foundation for further inquiry.

During the subsequent decade after the closure of RTOG 76-05, the RTOG initiated six additional trials for primary or metastatic liver malignancy. Five of the six trials used WLRT with various combinations of radiosensitizers, chemotherapies, radiopharmaceuticals, or alterations in the radiation delivery in attempts to improve the therapeutic benefit of RT. These strategies were pursued because radiation dose was limited by the radiosensitivity of the normal liver.[11,20-24] The standard radiation regimen for these studies was 21 Gy in 7 fractions.[20-22,24] In RTOG 80-03, patients were randomized to this regimen alone or in combination with misonidazole, a compound that selectively sensitizes hypoxic tumor cells to radiation. Although the addition of a

(*text continues on page 172*)

TABLE 9.2 Select Prospective Trials of Palliative RT to Liver

Study	Dose	Fields	Volume	Constraints	Effectiveness	Toxicity	Strength
Borgelt[8] N = 103, LM	Solitary: 3.04 Gy/19 fx 3 Gy/15 fx (optional 20 Gy boost) Multiple: 30 Gy/15 fx 25.6 Gy/16 fx 20 Gy/10 fx 21 Gy/7 fx	AP/PA, posterior block on left kidney (when possible)	Entire liver +2 cm margin; 1 cm margin for local boost to <1/3 of liver	Posterior block on kidney; boost volume to <1/3 of the liver	Improvements in eight different symptoms were reported with rates ranging from 19% to 55%; Abdominal pain, nausea/ vomiting, and fever had the highest improvement rates (55%, 49%, and 45%, respectively), Performance status improved in 25%	16% RT induced nausea/ vomiting, no documented cases of radiation hepatitis, nephritis, or pneumonitis	First cooperative group evaluation of palliative liver treatment, evaluated response in multiple symptoms, labs, performance status, and physical exam, large study

(continued)

TABLE 9.2 Select Prospective Trials of Palliative RT to Liver (*continued*)

Study	Dose	Fields	Volume	Constraints	Effectiveness	Toxicity	Strength
Leibel[21] *N* = 187, LM	21 Gy/7 fx Misonidazole given PO at 1.5 gm/m² daily 4–6 hr prior to RT	AP/PA opposed or oblique	Whole liver	Lower 2/3 of the left kidney was shielded or excluded from field	Misonidazole didn't improve therapeutic response in any tested parameter. Abd pain relieved in 80% (complete in 54%), prompt palliation with median time 1.7 wk with 13 wk duration of response, KPS improved in 28%, median OS was 4.2 m	22% developed nausea with 7% being severe, no RILD or nephritis, one case of RT pneumonitis requiring steroids. Misonidazole caused neuropathy in 20% of patients	Larger study confirming the benefits of WLRT for palliation of symptoms with little morbidity

(*continued*)

TABLE 9.2 Select Prospective Trials of Palliative RT to Liver (*continued*)

Study	Dose	Fields	Volume	Constraints	Effectiveness	Toxicity	Strength
Russell[11] N = 173, LM	Dose escalation 1.5 Gy BID to a total of 27 Gy, 30 Gy, or 33 Gy	Parallel opposed fields AP/PA or oblique	Whole liver, isocentric treatment, midplane depth, compensators encouraged to keep inhomogeneity ±10%	2/3rds of functional kidney needs to be excluded from field	Increasing WLRT dose didn't improve medial survival or decrease risk of death from liver metastases	Increased toxicity with higher dose, grade 3 toxicity seen only in 33 Gy group (11% acute, 33% late). In 33 Gy group, 10% risk of grade 3 radiation hepatitis at 6 months	Larger trial, suggested a higher safe liver dose threshold than was previously used

(*continued*)

TABLE 9.2 Select Prospective Trials of Palliative RT to Liver (*continued*)

Study	Dose	Fields	Volume	Constraints	Effectiveness	Toxicity	Strength
Bydder[3] *N* = 28 all LM, all symptomatic from liver lesion	10 Gy in 2 fx	AP/PA	Symptomatic portion of the liver +2 cm up to WL	Dose prescribed to midplane delivered 6–24 hr apart, block one kidney	Symptom response rates of 53%–66% at 2 wk, partial or complete symptomatic response in 54%	7% grade 3 toxicity (vomiting, diarrhea), 4 transient worsening of pain shortly after RT	Short course of treatment, limited toxicity with reasonable response
Soliman[14] *N* = 41, HCC (*N* = 21) or LM (*N* = 20)	8 Gy in 1 fx	AP/PA, oblique parallel opposed	Whole liver with at least 1 cm PTV margin	Target: 95% of the PTV to receive 7 Gy OAR: max dose of <10 Gy to stomach, small bowel, and spinal cord	48%–52% had improvement in symptoms at 1 month, improvements in FACT-G, EORTC GLG-C30 function and symptoms	Only two (7%) grade 3, low rate of grade 1-2 fatigue, nausea, and gastritis	Used validated patient-reported symptom and QoL questionnaires

AP/PA, anterior-posterior/posterior-anterior; fx, fraction; HCC, hepatocellular carcinoma; KPS, Karnofsky performance score; LM, liver metastases; OAR, organs at risk; QoL, quality of life; RILD, radiation-induced liver disease; RT, radiation therapy.

radiosensitizer didn't improve the therapeutic response in any of the tested parameters, the study confirmed the benefits of WLRT. In this cohort, 80% had their abdominal pain effectively palliated with 54% of these achieving complete remission. Palliation was relatively rapid with median time to relief of 1.7 weeks with a median duration of 13 weeks. For patients who lived 3 months, 52% maintained their improved pain status. Follow-up CT scans evaluated tumor response. Although the response was not robust by imaging criteria (0.6% complete response, 7% partial response, and 13% marginal response), patients still experienced symptomatic relief with the treatment.[21]

Investigations of chemotherapy and radiopharmaceuticals in addition to WLRT for primary liver tumors (RTOG 79-28, RTOG 83-01, RTOG 83-19), showed improved radiographic response by CT radiography compared to historical values (48% response rate with 7% complete and 41% partial), but there was increased toxicity and no survival benefit.[20,23-25]

An accelerated hyperfractionated study (RTOG 84-05) sought to determine if higher radiation doses could prolong survival and to gain a better understanding of liver tolerance to fractionated external beam radiation therapy. In this study, 173 patients with liver metastases from a primary GI site received 1.5 Gy twice a day to the whole liver with sequential groups receiving 27 Gy, 30 Gy, and 33 Gy total doses. This mild dose escalation did not prolong survival or decrease the rate of death from liver metastases, but five of the 51 patients entered on the 33 Gy group experienced late liver injury with an actuarial risk of severe radiation hepatitis (grade 3 or higher) of 10% at 6 months. Since no liver toxicity was observed in the 27 Gy and 30 Gy groups, this was thought to be a safe regimen.[11]

In addition to the previous studies using 21 Gy in 7 fractions as the standard dose for WLRT, two additional prospective trials investigated the effectiveness and tolerability of shorter radiation courses.[13,14] The first was a 28-patient cohort with symptomatic liver metastases treated with partial or whole liver irradiation of 10 Gy in 2 fractions given over 2 days. Individual symptom response rate for pain score, abdominal distention, night sweats, nausea, and vomiting were 53% to 66% at 2 weeks with partial or complete global symptomatic responses in 54% of treated patients. The majority (75%) of patients perceived benefit from the treatment. Toxicity was relatively limited with 7% experiencing grade 3 toxicity within 2 weeks of therapy (one episode of nausea, one episode of diarrhea) and 14% did have transient temporary increase in pain shortly after treatment.[13] The second study included 41 symptomatic patients with either primary or secondary liver malignancy who received 8 Gy to the whole liver in one fraction. One particular innovation of this study was the prospective utilization of the validated patient-reported symptoms and quality of life metrics [Brief Pain Index (BPI)], Functional Assessment of Cancer Therapy—Hepatobiliary (FACT-Hep), and the European Organization for Research and Treatment of Cancer Quality of Life Questionnaire C30 (EORTC QLQ-C30)). At one month, 48% had an improvement in symptoms. Improvements in the FACT-G and hepatobiliary subscale were seen in 23% to 29% of patients at 1 month. Improvements in EORTC QLQ-C30 functional (range 11%–21%) and symptom (range 11%–50 %) domains were also observed. Grade 3 toxicity was limited to one patient who declined premedication and developed nausea.[14] While these studies suggest useful palliation from short courses of whole liver irradiation, there are currently no published studies directly comparing any of the palliative whole liver radiation therapy regimens in a prospective randomized fashion. There is an ongoing phase III randomized trial by the National Cancer Institute of Canada (NCIC) HE1, of best supportive care compared to palliative radiation therapy for patients with HCC or liver metastases.

When managing patients with malignant liver disease with radiation therapy, the dose-limiting toxicity is usually RILD.[17,22,26] This has led to the development of low-dose WLRT as has been described. While this therapy can offer good palliation, the durability of local control, symptom palliation, and radiographic response may be limited. With the development of three-dimensional (3D) conformal radiation therapy, improvements in radiation therapy delivery techniques, and enhanced understanding of the partial tolerance of the liver to radiation therapy, ablative doses of radiation can safely be delivered to patients with limited liver disease with a potential for improved local control and durability of response. Initial efforts using 3D conformal radiation showed that even with high doses of radiation, the risk of RILD was low as long as the mean liver dose was in the range shown to be safe from the WLRT experiences (~30 Gy).[27] Several predictive models have been developed, which help estimate the risk of RILD.[28-30] These models use parameters like the whole liver dose associated with a 50% probability of toxicity; the volume of the liver receiving radiation, and even the type of malignancy to help predict if a given radiation plan is safe to deliver.

Greater understanding of the principles surrounding the partial volume tolerance of the liver to radiation coupled with improved visualization of liver tumors and more precise radiation therapy delivery techniques has led to the development of SBRT for liver tumors. This technique, which was initially developed for treating early stage lung cancer, uses increased conformity and steep dose gradients to deliver hypofractionated ablative doses to the target volume within the liver, while keeping the mean liver dose low and avoiding nearby critical structures. In comparison to WLRT, liver SBRT requires more complex treatment planning, more awareness, understanding, and management of organ motion (during and between treatments), more dependence on image guidance, more rigorous quality assurance and coordination, and increased cost, but has the potential for greater tumor control and improved treatment durability.[31] While WLRT is typically used in symptomatic patients with potentially widespread or multifocal liver and systemic disease, limited performance status, and relatively short survival potential, optimal patients for SBRT have limited liver and systemic disease, reasonable performance status, a potential for longer survival, and are typically asymptomatic from their liver malignancy. Several prospective trials have been conducted for both metastatic and primary liver lesions.[7,32] Overall, for liver metastases the 1-year local control ranges from 71% to 95% with limited reports of toxicity, and median survival rates of 17 to 20 months.[12,33-35] Likewise, prospective trials of SBRT for hepatocellular carcinoma yield similar high 1-year local control (75%–100%), limited toxicity, and reasonable 1-year overall survival rates of 55% to 75%.[36-39] Recent evidence also supports that SBRT causes no detriment to patient reported quality of life.[40]

One additional clinical situation where liver 3D conformal RT or SBRT may play an important role in palliation is in the case of HCC with portal vein thrombosis (PVT). PVT carries a poor prognosis with survival of only a few months without treatment. Many patients with PVT may not be eligible for standard therapies like surgery or radiofrequency ablation. There are multiple retrospective as well as several prospective studies evaluating 3D RT and SBRT in patients with PVT.[36,41-44] These studies suggest that radiation may improve vein patency and improve survival. The largest prospective study is from Princess Margaret Hospital, where they treated 56 patients with portal vein tumor thrombus with a 30 Gy to 54 Gy in 6 fractions regimen (median dose was 36 Gy in 6 fractions). They reported a 1-year overall survival rate of 44% with a median survival of almost 11 months.[36] Additional strategies for patients with PVT, for example, combining transarterial chemotherapy embolation (TACE) with radiation have shown promising 1- and 2-year overall survival rates of 42.5% and 22.8%.[44] Likewise a study investigating the addition of RT to percutaneous transhepatic portal vein stenting and TACE showed improved 1-year survival (32% vs. 6.9%, p < 0.01) for the patients receiving the additional RT.[43] Together, these data support the consideration of RT for patients with HCC and PVT.

Biliary obstruction caused from external compression of the bile duct or from tumor growing in the duct can be a significant cause of morbidity in patients with both primary and secondary liver malignancies. While biliary obstruction can be managed emergently through percutaneous drainage followed by conversion to internal stent or internal stent upfront in less emergent cases, external beam radiation may be helpful in select patients. Although the data is limited, some evidence suggests a benefit for adding radiation as a palliative measure to help keep stents patent longer or to help open externally compressed biliary ducts.[45-47]

In addition to the various forms of external beam radiation therapy, there is growing interest in radioembolization. This minimally invasive outpatient technique uses interventional radiological procedures to isolate the arterial supply of a liver tumor and selectively delivers radioactive material into the tumor vasculature. Yttrium-90 (Y-90) is the most commonly used isotope and can be attached to glass or resin beads. It is a pure-beta emitter with a half-life of about 64 hours and a tissue penetration range of 2.5 mm to 11 mm. With this technique, single or multiple tumors can be treated. Clinically, Y90 has been shown to slow progression and control both primary and secondary liver cancers.[48,49]

PLANNING

Simulation

Patients should be simulated supine with a CT scan with adequate immobilization to ensure reproducible set up with their arms above their heads. Estimates of respiratory motion should be acquired at time of simulation with either a 4D respiratory-correlated scan or inhalation/exhalation scans to get an approximation for organ movement. The degree of certainty regarding tumor and organ motion and rigidity for immobilization should reflect the intended radiation plan and technique, with patients undergoing SBRT or high-dose conformal treatments requiring more certainty than those being treated with low-dose whole liver treatments. Similarly, patients receiving more complex treatments may benefit from an MRI simulation, IV/oral contrast, or fiducial placement as part of the treatment planning process. Flouroscopic simulation may also be appropriate for WLRT to determine the degree of excursion of the liver with respiration, as it should be considered when designing treatment fields.

Target Delineation

Whole liver

For whole liver treatments, the gross tumor volume (GTV) should be defined as the area of the liver causing the symptoms. The clinical target volume (CTV) will be the entire liver with the planning target volume (PTV) representing a 1 cm to 2 cm margin around the CTV depending on the set up and immobilization of each patient. Organs at risk (OAR) (stomach, spinal cord, small and large bowel, and kidneys) should also be delineated on the simulation CT scan.

SBRT/high-dose 3D conformal

The GTV is defined by the tumor either on the planning CT or another fused diagnostic study (CT or MRI). For patients with significant motion of the GTV with respiration, a gated technique, active breathing control (ABC), or additional motion control (abdominal compression) is appropriate. For patients treated with a gated technique, the GTV should be delineated for only the phases of respiration when the beam will be on to create an internal tumor volume (ITV). For tumors with less respiratory movement due to position, abdominal compression, or active breath hold, the GTV should be delineated in the same manner as described, but the ITV should be created using all phases of the respiratory cycle. Patient-specific PTV margins ≥5 mm should be added to the ITV depending on patient and treatment factors including tumor respiratory motion, immobilization, and motion management strategy.

Treatment Plan

Whole liver

Three-dimensional planning should be used in order to understand the anatomy and guide field design and beam arrangements. Figure 9.1 shows a 3D WLRT plan. Typically, anterior-posterior opposed or oblique plans can be used based on the patient's anatomy and habitus to provide the best coverage of the whole liver while sparing radiation dose to the OAR. Megavoltage energy beams should be used. To avoid excessive dose to the kidneys, posterior blocks can be used to block the kidneys or they can be placed outside of the fields when possible. Excessively complicated plans should be avoided in severely symptomatic patients to avoid prolonged time on the treatment table. For tumor

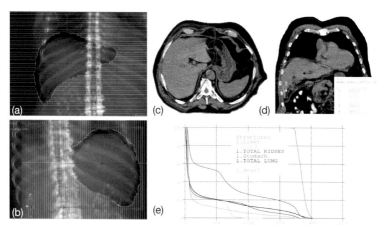

FIGURE 9.1 Radiation plan for whole liver external beam radiation therapy for a 65-year-old male with diffuse hepatic metastases causing abdominal pain. (a, b) Plan AP with a slight posterior oblique to partially avoid the right kidney. (c–e) Isodose lines and dose-volume histogram show coverage and the dose to surrounding organs.

coverage, the treatment goal of 95% of the PTV receiving a minimum of at least 90% of the prescribed dose should be adequate. The constraints for OARs are dependent on the dose to the whole liver and the fractionation. For 21 Gy in 3 Gy daily fractions, at least two-thirds of one kidney should be shielded or outside of the radiation field.[21] For 10 Gy in 5 Gy fractions, shielding of the kidney is recommended when possible and should be required for one kidney if both would be in the radiation field.[13] For 8 Gy in a single fraction, the maximum dose to the stomach, small bowel, and spinal cord must be less than 10 Gy.[14]

SBRT/High-dose 3D

3D planning should be used to determine beam arrangement and the most appropriate technique. Figure 9.2 shows a typical SBRT plan for a single liver metastasis. Techniques such as dynamic conformal arcs or multiple planar or noncoplanar beams (dynamic or static) with either 3D conformal or intensity modulated radiation therapy can be used. Beam energies should range from 6 to 18 MV. Efforts should be made to make treatment conformal to avoid excessive dose to the liver or surrounding structures. Constraints to OARs will vary slightly depending on the prescription dose and the number of fractions. Refer to Table 9.3 for suggested constraints.

Day of Treatment

Premedication

All patients should receive premedication with an oral antiemetic (ondansetron) and low dose dexamethasone about one hour prior to treatment. Patients with a substantial dose to the stomach or bowel may also benefit from an antacid to help reduce the risk of ulcer.

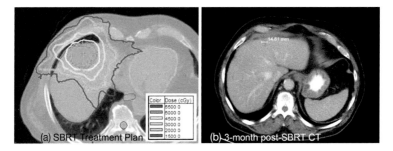

FIGURE 9.2 (a) SBRT plan for a 73-year-old male with a single 4.3 cm focus of metastatic melanoma to the liver. Treated with 50 Gy in 5 fractions. (b) Post-SBRT imaging at 3 months shows excellent tumor response with no observed acute toxicity.

TABLE 9.3 General Constraints for Liver SBRT

Liver (liver—GTV)	700 mL <15 Gy (3-fraction) for liver metastases
	Mean <13 Gy at 50 Gy in 5 fractions, for primary liver tumors, but mean dose may go up with smaller fraction sizes (mean of 17 for dose to 27.5 in 5 fractions)
Stomach	Max dose to 0.5 cc of 30 Gy
Small bowel/Duodenum	Max dose to 0.5 cc of 30 Gy
Large bowel	Max dose to 0.5 cc of 32 Gy
Esophagus	Max dose to 0.5 cc <30 Gy
Spinal cord + 5 mm	Max dose 25 Gy
Heart	Max dose to 0.5 cc <30 Gy
Kidney	bilateral mean dose <10 Gy
Bile duct	Avoid hot spots and long lengths of duct receiving high dose; max dose of 50 Gy
Chest wall	Max dose to 0.5 cc <50 Gy

GTV, gross tumor volume; SBRT, stereotactic body radiation therapy.

Image guidance

Prior to treatment, verification imaging should be performed to confirm the position of the liver and ensure proper coverage. For SBRT/high-dose 3D conformal treatments may require more intense verification imaging (cone beam CT, CT-on-rails, 4D cone beam, or gated verification CT) and motion management (respiratory monitoring during treatment).

Toxicity

Whole liver radiation therapy: WLRT is generally tolerated very well as long as the dose to the whole liver is limited to less than 30 Gy in 3 Gy fractions or 33 Gy in 1.5 BID fractions. Acute complications are uncommon. Transient fatigue can be seen in up to a third of patients.[14] Nausea is seen in less than 10% of patients and can be reduced with premedication.[8,13,14] A pain flare has been reported in about 14% of patients treated with 10 Gy in 5 Gy fractions, but premedication with steroids may also help reduce this number.[13] Risk of radiation hepatitis, pneumonitis, nephritis, or esophagitis is very rare with 21 Gy in 7 fractions, 10 Gy in 2 fractions, or 8 Gy in 1 fraction.

SBRT/High-dose 3D conformal: Generally, SBRT and high-dose 3D conformal radiation therapy is well tolerated in terms of acute and late toxicity for both metastases and primary liver tumors. Patients with primary liver tumors have a higher incidence of grade 3 to 5 toxicity, likely attributed to their poor liver reserves and underlying liver disease. Overall, the rate of grade ≥3 can range from 8% to 36% for primary liver tumors[36,38,39] and 2% to 10% for liver metastases.[12,33,34] One prospective study of advanced HCC reported grade 3, 4, and 5 toxicity rates of 26%, 3%, and 7%. The majority of the grade 3 toxicity were related to labs (11% elevated AST/ALT, and 9% decreased platelets). Five of the seven deaths were due to liver failure; the other deaths were due to cholangitis and a GI bleed.[36] GI bleeding can be severe and life-threatening when treating primary or secondary disease if lesions are close to stomach or bowel, but overall the reported rates of ≥3 grade toxicity are low.[12,34-36,38] Symptomatic chest wall toxicity has also been reported, but the incidence is less than 5%.[34]

Symptomatic improvement

Whole liver radiation therapy: WLRT improves symptoms in the majority of patients. Studies of WLRT for both primary and secondary liver malignancies show a palliative benefit in 49% to 95% of patients.[9-11,14,18,21] Improvement in pain is the most commonly reported benefit. Eighty percent of patients presenting with abdominal pain experience improvement in their symptoms with a complete response rate of 54%.[21] The median time to the amelioration of pain was 1.7 weeks following the start of WLRT.[21] Significant improvements in pain, abdominal distension, night sweats, nausea, and vomiting have been reported in greater than 50% of patients presenting with these symptoms.[13] Many will also experience improvements in their liver function tests (bilirubin, alkaline phosphatase, ALT/AST).[8,47] WLRT also increases Karnofsky performance status with a 10 to 20 point increase in about 25% of patients.[8,21]

SBRT/High-dose 3D conformal: Patients treated with these regimens are typically asymptomatic, so less data is available for improvement. Recent evidence suggests that these treatments have limited effect on quality of life.[40]

CLINICAL PEARLS

- Significant improvements in symptoms (pain, abdominal distension, night sweats, nausea, and vomiting) have been reported in greater than 50% of patients treated with palliative liver RT. Patients also experience improvements in liver function tests and Karnofsky performance scores.
- Common fractionation regimens include 21 Gy in 7 fractions, 10 Gy in 2 fractions, and 8 Gy in a single fraction.
- Palliation is relatively rapid (median time to relief of 1.7 weeks) and durable (median of 13 weeks).

SELF-ASSESSMENT

Questions

1. Which of the following are safe and appropriate doses for whole liver radiation therapy? (select all that apply)
   A. 21 Gy in 7 fractions
   B. 8 Gy in 1 fraction
   C. 33 Gy in 22 fractions delivered BID
   D. 10 Gy in 2 fractions

2. How can acute toxicity of liver irradiation be mitigated? (select all that apply)
   A. Premedication with an antiemetic about 1 hour prior to RT
   B. Premedication with dexamethasone prior to treatment
   C. Treating patients with full stomachs
   D. Giving BID fractions

3. Which of the following was the result of adding misonidazole, a selective radiosensitizer of hypoxic cells, to whole liver radiation therapy (RTOG 80-03)?
   A. Patients had superior palliation with improved symptoms and increased duration.
   B. Misonidazole did not significantly improve the frequency of any symptomatic palliation, complete pain response, the frequency of response, or overall survival.
   C. The median survival for patients treated with WLRT was 4.3 months compared to 6.5 months for WLRT + misonidazole.
   D. Patients treated with misonidazole did not have increased risk for developing peripheral neuropathy.

4. Which patient would be the best candidate for palliative whole liver radiation therapy?
   A. 55-year-old female with an asymptomatic single small liver lesion from a metastatic colorectal lesion in a peripheral location, with no other systemic disease and ECOG 0
   B. 75-year-year old male with multiple symptomatic large liver lesions from widely metastatic esophageal adenocarcinoma, ECOG 2
   C. 61-year-old male with multifocal asymptomatic HCC with Child-Pugh B cirrhosis from hepatitis C, ECOG 1
   D. 45-year old with new asymptomatic liver lesion and a history of colon cancer 3 years ago with no other evidence of disease. The liver lesion appears to be resectable, ECOG 0

5. When using SBRT to treat a liver metastasis, which of the following parameters would be considered safe?
   A. A mean liver dose (whole liver minus GTV) of 22 Gy
   B. Sparing at least 700 cc of the liver from more than 15 Gy
   C. Maximal dose to the small bowel of 37 Gy
   D. Max dose to cord + 0.5 cm of 30 Gy

Answers

1. A., B., D. Of the possible choices, only C. showed increased of liver toxicity.

2. A., B. Premedicating patient prior to liver RT reduces the risk of RT associated nausea and vomiting.

3. B. The results of RTOG 8003 showed no benefit adding misonidazole increased toxicity without providing significant clinical benefit.

4. B. Palliative WLRT is best delivered to a symptomatic patient. Patients with limited asymptomatic may be eligible for other liver-directed therapies with better potential for durable response.

5. B. This was one of the dosimetric guidelines for liver metastases used by Rustoven et al.[43] The other parameters would typically not be considered safe.

REFERENCES

1. Siegel RL, Miller KD, Jemal A. Cancer statistics, 2015. *CA Cancer J Clin*. 2015;65(1):5-29.
2. Ananthakrishnan A, Gogineni V, Saeian K. Epidemiology of primary and secondary liver cancers. *Semin Intervent Radiol*. 2006;23(1):47-63.
3. American Cancer Society. *Global Cancer Facts & Figures*. 3rd ed. Atlanta, GA: American Cancer Society; 2015.
4. Yeung YP, Lo CM, Liu CL, et al. Natural history of untreated nonsurgical hepatocellular carcinoma. *Am J Gastroenterol*. 2005;100(9):1995-2004.
5. Okuda K, Ohtsuki T, Obata H, et al. Natural history of hepatocellular carcinoma and prognosis in relation to treatment. Study of 850 patients. *Cancer*. 1985;56(4):918-928.
6. Dhir M, Lyden ER, Smith LM, Are C. Comparison of outcomes of transplantation and resection in patients with early hepatocellular carcinoma: a meta-analysis. *HPB (Oxford)*. 2012;14(9):635-645.
7. Tanguturi SK, Wo JY, Zhu AX, et al. Radiation therapy for liver tumors: ready for inclusion in guidelines? *The Oncologist*. 2014;19(8):868-879.
8. Borgelt BB, Gelber R, Brady LW, et al. The palliation of hepatic metastases: results of the Radiation Therapy Oncology Group pilot study. *Int J Radiat Oncol Biol Phys*. 1981;7(5):587-591.

9. Phillips R, Karnofsky DA, Hamilton LD, Nickson JJ. Roentgen therapy of hepatic metastases. *Am J Roentgenol Radium Ther Nucl Med.* 1954;71(5):826-834.

10. Prasad B, Lee MS, Hendrickson FR. Irradiation of hepatic metastases. *Int J Radiat Oncol Biol Phys.* 1977;2(1-2):129-132.

11. Russell AH, Clyde C, Wasserman TH, et al. Accelerated hyperfractionated hepatic irradiation in the management of patients with liver metastases: results of the RTOG dose escalating protocol. *Int J Radiat Oncol Biol Phys.* 1993;27(1);117-123.

12. Hoyer M, Roed H, Traberg Hansen A, et al. Phase II study on stereotactic body radiotherapy of colorectal metastases. *Acta Oncol.* 2006;45(7):823-830.

13. Bydder S, Spry NA, Christie DR, et al. A prospective trial of short-fractionation radiotherapy for the palliation of liver metastases. *Australas Radiol.* 2003;47(3):284-288.

14. Soliman H, Ringash J, Jiang H, et al. Phase II trial of palliative radio-therapy for hepatocellular carcinoma and liver metastases. *J Clin Oncol.* 2013;31(31):3980-3986.

15. Cunningham SC, Choti MA, Bellavance EC, Pawlik TM. Palliation of hepatic tumors. *Surg Oncol.* 2007;16(4):277-291.

16. Turek M. Radiation therapy of the liver metastatic disease. *Radiol Clin.* 1975;44(2):142-145.

17. Ingold JA, Reed GB, Kaplan HS, Bagshaw MA. Radiation Hepatitis. *Am J Roentgenol Radium Ther Nucl Med.* 1965;93:200-208.

18. Sherman DM, Weichselbaum R, Order SE, et al. Palliation of hepatic metastasis. *Cancer.* 1978;41(5):2013-2017.

19. Stearns MW, Jr., Leaming RH. Irradiation in inoperable cancer. *JAMA.* 1975;231(13):1388.

20. Abrams RA, Pajak TF, Haulk TL, et al. Survival results among patients with alpha-fetoprotein-positive, unresectable hepatocellular carcinoma: analysis of three sequential treatments of the RTOG and Johns Hopkins Oncology Center. *Cancer J Sci Am.* 1998;4(3):178-184.

21. Leibel SA, Pajak TF, Massullo V, et al. A comparison of misonidazole sensitized radiation therapy to radiation therapy alone for the palliation of hepatic metastases: results of a Radiation Therapy Oncology Group randomized prospective trial. *Int J Radiat Oncol Biol Phys.* 1987;13(7):1057-1064.

22. Leibel SA, Guse C, Order SE, et al. Accelerated fractionation radiation therapy for liver metastases: selection of an optimal patient population for the evaluation of late hepatic injury in RTOG studies. *Int J Radiat Oncol Biol Phys.* 1990;18(3):523-528.

23. Ettinger DS, Order SE, Wharam MD, et al. Phase I-II study of isotopic immunoglobulin therapy for primary liver cancer. *Cancer Treat Rep.* 1982;66(2):289-297.

24. Order S, Pajak T, Leibel S, et al. A randomized prospective trial comparing full dose chemotherapy to 131I antiferritin: an RTOG study. *Int J Radiat Oncol Biol Phys.* 1991;20(5):953-963.

25. Order SE, Stillwagon GB, Klein JL, et al. Iodine 131 antiferritin, a new treatment modality in hepatoma: a Radiation Therapy Oncology Group study. *J Clin Oncol*. 1985;3(12):1573-1582.
26. Lawrence TS, Robertson JM, Anscher MS, et al. Hepatic toxicity resulting from cancer treatment. *Int J Radiat Oncol Biol Phys*. 1995;31(5):1237-1248.
27. Dawson LA, Normolle D, Balter JM, et al. Analysis of radiation-induced liver disease using the Lyman NTCP model. *Int J Radiat Oncol Biol Phys*. 2002;53(4):810-821.
28. McGinn CJ, Ten Haken RK, Ensminger WD, et al. Treatment of intrahepatic cancers with radiation doses based on a normal tissue complication probability model. *J Clin Oncol*. 1998;16(6):2246-2252.
29. Dawson LA, Ten Haken RK. Partial volume tolerance of the liver to radiation. *Semin Radiat Oncol*. 2005;15(4):279-283.
30. Cozzi L, Buffa FM, Fogliata A. Comparative analysis of dose volume histogram reduction algorithms for normal tissue complication probability calculations. *Acta Oncol*. 2000;39(2):165-171.
31. Potters L, Kavanagh B, Galvin JM, et al. American Society for Therapeutic Radiology and Oncology (ASTRO) and American College of Radiology (ACR) practice guideline for the performance of stereotactic body radiation therapy. *Int J Radiat Oncol Biol Phys*. 2010;76(2):326-332.
32. Hoyer M, Swaminath A, Bydder S, et al. Radiotherapy for liver metastases: a review of evidence. *Int J Radiat Oncol Biol Phys*. 2012;82(3):1047-1057.
33. Herfarth KK, Debus J, Wannenmacher M. Stereotactic radiation therapy of liver metastases: update of the initial phase-I/II trial. *Front Radiat Ther Oncol*. 2004;38:100-105.
34. Rusthoven KE, Kavanagh BD, Cardenes H, et al. Multi-institutional phase I/II trial of stereotactic body radiation therapy for liver metastases. *J Clin Oncol*. 2009;27(10):1572-1578.
35. Lee MT, Kim JJ, Dinniwell R, et al. Phase I study of individualized stereotactic body radiotherapy of liver metastases. *J Clin Oncol*. 2009;27(10):1585-1591.
36. Bujold A, Massey CA, Kim JJ, et al. Sequential phase I and II trials of stereotactic body radiotherapy for locally advanced hepatocellular carcinoma. *J Clin Oncol*. 2013;31(13):1631-1639.
37. Kang JK, Kim MS, Cho CK, et al. Stereotactic body radiation therapy for inoperable hepatocellular carcinoma as a local salvage treatment after incomplete transarterial chemoembolization. *Cancer*. 2012;118(21):5424-5431.
38. Cardenes HR, Price TR, Perkins SM, et al. Phase I feasibility trial of stereotactic body radiation therapy for primary hepatocellular carcinoma. *Clinical Transl Oncol*. 2010;12(3):218-225.
39. Tse RV, Hawkins M, Lockwood G, et al. Phase I study of individualized stereotactic body radiotherapy for hepatocellular carcinoma and intrahepatic cholangiocarcinoma. *J Clin Oncol*. 2008;26(4):657-664.
40. Klein J, Dawson LA, Jiang H, et al. Prospective longitudinal assessment of quality of life for liver cancer patients treated with stereotactic body radiation therapy. *Int J Radiat Oncol Biol Phys*. 2015;93(1):16-25.

41. Yeh SA, Chen YS, Perng DS. The role of radiotherapy in the treatment of hepatocellular carcinoma with portal vein tumor thrombus. *J Radiat Res.* 2015;56(2):325-331.

42. Zeng ZC, Fan J, Tang ZY, et al. A comparison of treatment combinations with and without radiotherapy for hepatocellular carcinoma with portal vein and/or inferior vena cava tumor thrombus. *Int J Radiat Oncol Biol Phys.* 2005;61(2):432-443.

43. Zhang XB, Wang JH, Yan ZP, et al. Hepatocellular carcinoma with main portal vein tumor thrombus: treatment with 3-dimensional conformal radiotherapy after portal vein stenting and transarterial chemoembolization. *Cancer.* 2009;115(6):1245-1252.

44. Yoon SM, Lim YS, Won HJ, et al. Radiotherapy plus transarterial chemoembolization for hepatocellular carcinoma invading the portal vein: long-term patient outcomes. *Int J Radiat Oncol Biol Phys.* 2012;82(5):2004-2011.

45. Kuvshinoff BW, Armstrong JG, Fong Y, et al. Palliation of irresectable hilar cholangiocarcinoma with biliary drainage and radiotherapy. *Br J Surg.* 1995;82(11):1522-1525.

46. Ohnishi H, Asada M, Shichijo Y, et al. External radiotherapy for biliary decompression of hilar cholangiocarcinoma. *Hepato-gastroenterology.* 1995;42(3):265-268.

47. Yeo SG, Kim DY, Kim TH, et al. Whole-liver radiotherapy for end-stage colorectal cancer patients with massive liver metastases and advanced hepatic dysfunction. *Radiat Oncol.* 2010;5:97.

48. Habib A, Desai K, Hickey R, et al. Transarterial approaches to primary and seconadary hepatic malignancies. *Nat Rev Oncol.* 2015;12(8):481-489.

49. Memon K, Lewandowski RJ, Kulik L, et al. Radioembolization for primary and metastatic liver cancer. *Semin Radiat Oncol.* 2011;12(4):294-302.

Appendix A

These are general dose guidelines based on the literature presented in the text. Depending on the specific patient and planning approach, some fractionation schemes may be more appropriate than others with respect to normal tissue constraints and the patient's life expectancy. For additional details, refer to the chapter text and the primary literature supporting the dose fractionation scheme.

TABLE A.1 Palliative Radiation Fractionation Schemes for Bone Metastasis

Prognosis	Treatment Options
<1 month	■ Supportive care ■ Single 8 Gy fraction RT
>1 month	■ Supportive care ■ Single 8 Gy fraction RT ■ Consider higher dose (20–30 Gy in 5–10 fractions) for complicated bone metastasis
>1 month with risk of fracture*	■ Supportive care ■ Single 8 Gy fraction RT ■ Consider higher dose (20–30 Gy in 5–10 fractions) for complicated bone metastasis ■ Consideration of surgical stabilization with postoperative RT
Recurrent pain after initial course	■ Supportive Care ■ Single 8 Gy fraction

RT, radiation therapy.

*Based on Mirel's criteria or longest axial diameter of cortical involvement.

TABLE A.2 Palliative Radiation Fractionation Schemes for Spinal Cord Compression

Prognosis	Treatment Options
<3 months	■ Supportive care ■ Single 8 Gy fraction RT ■ 16 Gy in 2 fractions one week apart

>3 months
Not a surgical candidate
	■ Supportive care
	■ Short course RT
	  ■ 20 Gy in 5 fractions
	  ■ 30 Gy in 10 fractions

>3 months
Surgical candidate
	■ Supportive care
	■ Surgical decompression
	■ Postoperative RT
	  ■ 20 Gy in 5 fractions
	  ■ 30 Gy in 10 fractions

RT, radiation therapy.

TABLE A.3 Palliative Radiation Fractionation Schemes for Brain Metastasis

Prognosis	Treatment Options
<1 month	■ Supportive care ■ Steroids alone ■ Short course RT ■ 20 Gy in 5 fractions

>1 month
Multiple brain metastasis
All <4 cm
	■ Supportive care
	■ SRS
	■ WBRT
	  ■ 20 Gy in 5 fractions
	  ■ 30 Gy in 10 fractions
	■ WBRT ± SRS

>1 month
Multiple brain metastasis
At least one >4 cm
	■ Supportive care
	■ WBRT
	  ■ 20 Gy in 5 fractions
	  ■ 30 Gy in 10 fractions

>1 month
Solitary brain metastasis
	■ Surgical resection
	■ SRS
	■ ± WBRT
	  ■ 20 Gy in 5 fractions
	  ■ 30 Gy in 10 fractions

RT, radiation therapy; SRS, stereotactic radiosurgery; WBRT, whole brain radiation therapy.

TABLE A.4 Palliative Radiation Fractionation Schemes for Head and Neck Cancers

Prognosis	Treatment Options
<3 months	<ul><li>Supportive care</li><li>8 Gy repeated up to 3 times at weekly intervals to a dose of 24 Gy</li><li>17 Gy in 2 fractions of 8.5 Gy, 1 week apart</li></ul>
3–9 months	<ul><li>Supportive care</li><li>3.7 Gy BID x4 with ≥6 hour inter-fraction interval, repeated monthly up to 3 times, to a total dose of 44.4 Gy</li></ul>
>9 months	<ul><li>Supportive care</li><li>50 Gy in 25 fractions</li></ul>

BID, twice per day.

TABLE A.5 Palliative Radiation Fractionation Schemes for Lung Tumors

Prognosis	Treatment Options
<1 month	<ul><li>Supportive care</li><li>8–10 Gy in a single fraction</li><li>17 Gy in 2 fractions of 8.5 Gy, 1 week apart</li></ul>
>1 month	<ul><li>Supportive care</li><li>17 Gy in 2 fractions of 8.5 Gy, 1 week apart</li><li>30–39 Gy at 3 Gy per fraction</li></ul>

TABLE A.6 Palliative Radiation Fractionation Schemes for Abdominopelvic tumors

Prognosis	Treatment Options
<1 month	<ul><li>Supportive care</li><li>8–10 Gy x 1 or 2 with at least 1 week between fractions</li></ul>
>1 month	<ul><li>Supportive care</li><li>8–10 Gy x 1 or 2 with at least 1 week between fractions</li><li>20–30 Gy in 4–6 fractions</li><li>18–24 Gy in 3 fractions at weekly intervals</li></ul>
Frail patients with poor KPS and otherwise curable disease	<ul><li>Supportive care</li><li>20–25 Gy in 4–5 fractions</li><li>18–21 Gy in 3 fractions at weekly intervals</li></ul>

KPS, Karnofsky performance score.

TABLE A.7 Palliative Radiation Fractionation Schemes for Liver Tumors

Prognosis	Treatment Options
<3 months	■ Supportive care ■ Whole or partial liver: Single 8 Gy fraction RT or 10 Gy in 2 fractions
4–6 months	■ Supportive care ■ Whole liver: 21 Gy in 7 fractions ■ Whole or partial liver: Single 8 Gy fraction RT or 10 Gy in 2 fractions
6–12 months	■ Supportive care ■ Whole liver: 21 Gy in 7 fractions ■ Partial liver RT with dose respective of liver and tissue tolerance, such as 36 Gy in 6 fractions ■ Liver only disease may consider SBRT or high-dose 3D depending on situation
>1 year	■ Supportive care ■ SBRT 35–60 Gy in 3–5 fractions ■ High dose 3D conformal RT

RT, radiation therapy; SBRT, stereotactic body radiation therapy.

Appendix B

TABLE B.1 Tools to Help Assess Life Expectancy in Patients With Advanced Cancer

Tool (References)	Factors Incorporated	Comment
National Hospice Study[1]	KPS Anorexia Weight loss Dyspnea Dry mouth Dysphagia	Based on hospice patients If KPS ≥50 and none of five factors, median survival 6 months; with all five factors, 6 weeks.
Palliative Performance Scale[2]	Ambulatory status Activity level Disease status Self-care Intake Consciousness	Correlated with survival Applicable to cancer populations
Palliative Prognostic Index[3,4]	KPS Dyspnea at rest Oral intake Edema Delirium	Short-term survival of terminally ill cancer patients
Palliative Prognostic Score[5]	KPS Anorexia, dyspnea High total WBC Low lymphocyte percent Clinician's prediction of survival (weeks)	Valid for terminally ill or advanced cancer patients
Terminal Cancer Prognostic Scale[6]	Anorexia Diarrhea Confusion	Patients no longer receiving anticancer therapy
Taiwanese Scale[7]	Metastatic site KPS Symptoms Clinical signs	Predicts very short-term survival

(*continued*)

TABLE B.1 Tools to Help Assess Life Expectancy in Patients With Advanced Cancer (*continued*)

Tool (References)	Factors Incorporated	Comment
SUPPORT Model[8]	Physiology score day 3 Glasgow Coma Scale Score Age Disease class Length of hospital stay Cancer as comorbidity	Applies to very ill hospitalized patients
Glasgow Prognosis Score[9,10]	Albumin C-reactive protein	Terminally ill cancer patients
CRP-Vitamin B_{12} Product[11]	Vitamin B_{12} level C-reactive protein	Terminally ill cancer patients
Prognosis in Palliative Care Study[12,13]	KPS Mental test score Selected laboratory values Selected symptoms Primary site Site of metastasis	Predicts 2 weeks and 2 months survival Prognostic with or without lab values

CRP, C-reactive protein; KPS, Karnofsky performance score.

REFERENCES

1. Rees GJ, Devrell CE, Barley VL, Newman HF. Palliative radiotherapy for lung cancer: two versus five fractions. *Clin Oncol (R Coll Radiol)*. 1997;9(2): 90-95. PubMed PMID: 9135893.

2. Anderson F, Downing GM, Hill J, Casorso L, Lerch N. Palliative performance scale (PPS): a new tool. *J Palliat Care*. Spring 1996;12(1):5-11. PubMed PMID: 8857241.

3. Morita T, Tsunoda J, Inoue S, Chihara S. Validity of the palliative performance scale from a survival perspective. *J Pain Symptom Manage*. July 1999;18(1): 2-3. PubMed PMID: 10439564.

4. Morita T, Tsunoda J, Inoue S, Chihara S. Survival prediction of terminally ill cancer patients by clinical symptoms: development of a simple indicator. *Jpn J Clin Oncol*. March 1999;29(3):156-159. PubMed PMID: 10225699.

5. Pirovano M, Maltoni M, Nanni O, et al. A new palliative prognostic score: a first step for the staging of terminally ill cancer patients. Italian

Multicenter and Study Group on Palliative Care. *J Pain Symptom Manage.* April 1999;17(4):231-239. PubMed PMID: 10203875.

6. Yun YH, Heo DS, Heo BY, Yoo TW, Bae JM, Ahn SH. Development of terminal cancer prognostic score as an index in terminally ill cancer patients. *Oncol Rep*. July–August 2001;8(4):795-800. PubMed PMID: 11410786.

7. Chuang RB, Hu WY, Chiu TY, Chen CY. Prediction of survival in terminal cancer patients in Taiwan: constructing a prognostic scale. *J Pain Symptom Manage*. August 2004;28(2):115-122. PubMed PMID: 15276192.

8. Knaus WA, Harrell FE Jr., Lynn J, et al. The SUPPORT prognostic model. Objective estimates of survival for seriously ill hospitalized adults. Study to understand prognoses and preferences for outcomes and risks of treatments. *Ann Intern Med*. February 1, 1995;122(3):191-203. PubMed PMID: 7810938.

9. Elahi MM, McMillan DC, McArdle CS, Angerson WJ, Sattar N. Score based on hypoalbuminemia and elevated C-reactive protein predicts survival in patients with advanced gastrointestinal cancer. *Nutr Cancer*. 2004;48(2): 171-173. PubMed PMID: 15231451.

10. Forrest LM, McMillan DC, McArdle CS, Angerson WJ, Dunlop DJ. Evaluation of cumulative prognostic scores based on the systemic inflammatory response in patients with inoperable non-small-cell lung cancer. *Br J Cancer*. September 15, 2003;89(6):1028-1030. PubMed PMID: 12966420. Pubmed Central PMCID: 2376960.

11. Geissbuhler P, Mermillod B, Rapin CH. Elevated serum vitamin B_{12} levels associated with CRP as a predictive factor of mortality in palliative care cancer patients: a prospective study over five years. *J Pain Symptom Manage*. August 2000;20(2):93-103. PubMed PMID: 10989247.

12. Gwilliam B, Keeley V, Todd C, et al. Development of prognosis in palliative care study (PiPS) predictor models to improve prognostication in advanced cancer: prospective cohort study. *BMJ*. 2011;343:d4920. PubMed PMID: 21868477. Pubmed Central PMCID: 3162041.

13. Prognosis in Palliative Care Study Prognosticator [cited 2014 September 12]. Available at: http://www.pips.sgul.ac.uk/index.htm.

Index

Printed in the United States
By Bookmasters